SpringerBriefs in Public Health

Child Health

Series editor
Angelo P. Giardino, Houston, TX, USA

SpringerBriefs in Public Health present concise summaries of cutting-edge research and practical applications from across the entire field of public health, with contributions from medicine, bioethics, health economics, public policy, biostatistics, and sociology.

The focus of the series is to highlight current topics in public health of interest to a global audience, including health care policy; social determinants of health; health issues in developing countries; new research methods; chronic and infectious disease epidemics; and innovative health interventions.

Featuring compact volumes of 50 to 125 pages, the series covers a range of content from professional to academic. Possible volumes in the series may consist of timely reports of state-of-the art analytical techniques, reports from the field, snapshots of hot and/or emerging topics, elaborated theses, literature reviews, and in-depth case studies. Both solicited and unsolicited manuscripts are considered for publication in this series.

Briefs are published as part of Springer's eBook collection, with millions of users worldwide. In addition, Briefs are available for individual print and electronic purchase.

Briefs are characterized by fast, global electronic dissemination, standard publishing contracts, easy-to-use manuscript preparation and formatting guidelines, and expedited production schedules. We aim for publication 8–12 weeks after acceptance.

More information about this series at http://www.springer.com/series/11600

Rosina Avila Connelly • Teri Turner
Editors

Health Literacy and Child Health Outcomes

Promoting Effective Health Communication
Strategies to Improve Quality of Care

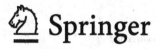
Springer

Editors
Rosina Avila Connelly
Department of Pediatrics & Adolescent
    Medicine, Division of General Pediatrics
University of South Alabama
Mobile, AL, USA

Teri Turner
Department of Pediatrics
Baylor College of Medicine/Texas Children's
    Hospital
Houston, TX, USA

ISSN 2192-3698   ISSN 2192-3701   (electronic)
SpringerBriefs in Public Health
ISBN 978-3-319-50798-9   ISBN 978-3-319-50799-6   (eBook)
DOI 10.1007/978-3-319-50799-6

Library of Congress Control Number: 2017934877

Printed on acid-free paper

This Springer imprint is published by Springer Nature
The registered company is Springer International Publishing AG
The registered company address is: Gewerbestrasse 11, 6330 Cham, Switzerland

Foreword

This monograph is just what pediatricians baffled by miscommunication have been looking for. It gives data on prevalence of low health literacy, briefly reviews the pediatric literature on the impact of low health literacy on child health outcomes, and offers practical strategies for the busy pediatrician.

Pediatricians love to care for children and want the best health care for all their patients. They value providing anticipatory guidance and giving parents needed instructions about medications, inhaler use, healthy eating etc. However they often fail to grasp the wide chasm that separates what they say and what parents actually understand and can act on. Patients with low health literacy struggle to understand and use health information and services. Sometimes parents may be too embarrassed to ask questions during the visit. At other times, like hospital discharge, parents may believe they have understood instructions and not realize until they get home that they are not clear how to manage a problem or whom to call.

The NIH's view on health communication indicates we must not blame individuals for not understanding information that has not been made clear to them. The NIH points out that everyone, no matter how well educated, is at risk for misunderstanding health information. This is especially true if the issue is emotionally charged, the instructions are complex, or a parent is anxious, distracted, or their child is sick.

Health information and services are becoming more complex and there are a rapidly increasing number of prescription and over-the-counter medications available. Parents can easily become confused and overwhelmed and unintentionally dose their child incorrectly. It is also increasingly difficult for young parents to separate evidence-based health information online and in places like "mommy blogs" from misleading or false information.

Parents and age-appropriate pediatric patients must become more fully engaged. To encourage their engagement, providers and health systems need to be more patient-centered and user-friendly. We are the ones who must take the initiative in making written and oral information easier to understand and use and not place the burden solely on parents to understand information that is not clear to them.

This brief monograph gives pediatricians reliable, evidence-based information on what they need to know about low health literacy as well as easy-to-use strategies for using plain language verbally and in written health materials and forms. The authors wisely suggest adopting at least one health literacy strategy such as avoiding jargon, limiting information, or asking patients/parents to teach back or show back to confirm their understanding. They offer a plan to improve communication without increasing time by following the "universal precautions" principle of giving all parents brief, to-the-point, concrete, and specific information focused on what they need to know and do, and pointing out the benefits.

Terry Davis

Terry C. Davis
Feist-Weiller Cancer Center Faculty
Department of Medicine and Pediatrics
LSU Health Sciences Center
Shreveport, LA, USA

Preface

This book was written and co-edited by a group of academic pediatricians who share the common passion for health literacy. Our group strives for disseminating our scholarly interest in many capacities. We want others to understand the important role that health literacy plays in effective health communication and child health outcomes. Thank you for your interest in reading our work.

A Google search for *"health literacy and child health outcomes"* yielded exactly 3,070,000 results in 0.47 s as of June 12, 2016—a vast amount of information for anyone to fathom. Especially if hearing these terms for the very first time, or for anyone seeking to learn more about the topic. It takes 0.47 min or less to read through the end of the next paragraph. We hope to interest the readers to look into the rest of this monograph.

Health literacy is an important determinant of health. It influences effective health communication, patient satisfaction, and patient safety. It impacts quality of care and health outcomes, health disparities, and quality of life. Low health literacy costs millions of dollars in extra health care costs. And low health literacy affects more American adults—and children—than one would begin to imagine.

In this book readers will find relevant and practical information on the subject of health literacy and child health outcomes, including communication strategies to use where the rubber meets the road. Strategies that might take less than 4.7 min to implement, but will result in exponential improvements in health. All packed in fewer than 150 pages of our double-spaced, 12-point font Times New Roman manuscript.

Our goal is to promote effective health communication to improve pediatric quality of care. We truly hope to advance the readers' knowledge and interest in health literacy and child health outcomes.

We thank you for your interest and time.

Sincerely,

Mobile, AL, USA
Houston, TX, USA

Rosina Avila Connelly
Teri Turner

Acknowledgments

The authors wish to express their appreciation to:

- Alejandro Torres, BA, who assisted in reviewing and editing of Chap. 3 on Medical Errors
- Betty "Lee" Ligon, PhD, MA, MAR, from the Center for Research, Innovation, and Scholarship in Medical Education at Texas Children's Hospital for her editorial assistance
- Janet Kim, MPH, Editor, Public Health at Springer, for her consistent encouragement to produce this monograph on Health Literacy and offering it as part of the Child Health Series

Contents

Chapter 1
Health Literacy and Health Communication

Rosina Avila Connelly and Michael E. Speer

> *To effectively communicate, we must realize that we are*
> *all different in the way we perceive the world and use this*
> *understanding as a guide to our communication with others.*
>
> –Tony Robbins

Imagine going to a restaurant in a different country and being unable to understand the server or the menu. In the interest of time, the server recommends you order the house's special entrée, as it is the best option on the menu and what most people enjoy, but does not stop to consider dietary food preferences, allergies, or special dietary needs. When your food arrives, you may eat it and enjoy it: all is well, and you leave satisfied, with plans to return to the restaurant in the future. Or … you may try it and not like it; you may find it unappealing and not even touch it. You pay the bill and leave with the intention of never returning to this restaurant; further, you are still hungry and so you go somewhere else to eat. Or, you may eat it and get ill, spend more money for medical treatments, lose time from work or leisure, and end up being very upset with the server, the restaurant, and, perhaps, yourself. Would it not have been a much more pleasant and cost-effective experience had the server spoken English? Would it not have been easier had the menu provided English translations, pictures, and warnings … or had the server confirmed that you understood what you were ordering? For that matter, did anyone even ask you if you cared to go to that particular restaurant?

R.A. Connelly (✉)
Division of General Pediatrics, Department of Pediatrics and Adolescent Medicine,
University of South Alabama, Mobile, AL, USA
e mail: rosinaconnelly@health.southalabama.edu

M.E. Speer, M.D.
Professor of Pediatrics and Ethics, Section of Neonatology, Department of Pediatrics,
Baylor College of Medicine, Texas Children's Hospital, Houston, TX, USA

© The Editor(s) and The Author(s) 2017
R.A. Connelly, T. Turner (eds.), *Health Literacy and Child Health Outcomes*,
SpringerBriefs in Public Health, DOI 10.1007/978-3-319-50799-6_1

Health Communication

"The single biggest problem with communication is the illusion that it has taken place."

—George Bernard Shaw

Communication is defined as *"the act or process of using words, sounds, signs, or behaviors to express or exchange information or to express your ideas, thoughts, feeling, etc., to someone else"* [1].

In medicine, good communication skills can result in greater patient satisfaction and compliance with medical treatments, improved health outcomes, decreased healthcare costs, and fewer malpractice claims [2–4]. Good communication skills are essential for interacting with patients and for providing effective health care [2]. In addition to communication skills, there are three elements that impact health communication. The Joint Commission described limited English proficiency, cultural differences, and low health literacy as the "triple threat" to effective health communication and patient safety, and it urges clinicians and organizations to address this triple threat in order to improve the safety and quality of patient care [5].

This monograph presents practical information relating to Health Literacy in the context of child health. We compile simple strategies to address the barriers regarding health literacy; by presenting health information such that patients can understand it and checking to ensure that communication did occur, clinicians caring for children can advance effective health communication and pediatric quality care [6].

Health Literacy

"Literacy unlocks the door to learning throughout life, is essential to development and health, and opens the way for democratic participation and active citizenship."

—Kofi Annan

In December 2006, in reference to this costly public health problem, Rear Admiral Kenneth P. Moritsugu, MD, MPH, Acting United States Surgeon General, said it is *"…a threat to the health and wellbeing of Americans…crosses all sectors of our society. All ages, races, incomes and education levels are challenged by [it]…"* [7].

If this were the information given, as an answer on the popular game show on national television "Jeopardy", the correct question would be *'What is low health literacy?'*

For practical purposes, health literacy is one of the key elements in Health Communication: one must be able to understand health information in order to have effective communication related to health.

What Is 'Health Literacy' and How Do We Know It Is 'Low'?

"There are all kinds of things you can do to marry literacy with health"

—C. Everett Koop, MD

A simple definition of 'Literacy' is "the ability to read and write" [8]. The 2003 National Assessment of Adult Literacy takes the simple definition of 'Literacy' to the twenty-first century level: the knowledge and skills necessary to perform literacy tasks [9]. Literacy means being able to acquire information using prose, document and quantitative skills, understand the information, and apply it to our daily lives. Another simple definition of *'Literacy'* is *"knowledge that relates to a specified subject"* [8].

'Health Literacy,' then, is simply the knowledge that relates to the subject of health, especially as it concerns healthy living. The Institute of Medicine has formally defined it as "the degree to which individuals have the capacity to obtain, process, and understand basic health information and services needed to make appropriate health decisions" [10].

> *"An ounce of prevention is worth a pound of cure."*
>
> —American Idiom

Universal Precautions

There are many ways to measure health literacy at the individual level, which are discussed later in other chapters in this book: patients' health literacy level, providers' use of health literacy skills, how health literacy-friendly are the institutions, and the complexity of the medical information and the system as a whole [11].

Limited health literacy skills are commonplace, we do not know easily, just by looking at the patients and their families. Therefore, the issue of low health literacy skills should be approached in a similar manner as the "universal precautions approach". It is not realistic to formally assess our patients' health literacy skills in every encounter. We do not stop to check any bodily fluid for infectious agents; we use the Universal Precautions approach and treat everything as potentially infectious [12]. Anyone could have difficulties managing health information under stressful situations; therefore we should approach health literacy the same way and utilize the "Health Literacy Universal Precautions" [13].

> *"Common sense is not so common."*
>
> —Voltaire

For those of us in the medical field *basic health information needed to make appropriate health decisions* would be just *"common sense"* as defined in the Merriam-Webster Dictionary: *'sound and prudent judgment based on a simple perception of the situation or facts'* [14].

As pediatricians, taking care of children's basic health problems is *'common sense'!* Contrariwise, the anxious first-time mother with a baby who awakens in the middle of the night, crying, has chills because of high fever, and is vomiting may not have the "common sense" to get fever-reducing medicine, read the instructions, measure the right amount of medicine with the dropper, and comfort her baby.

"All mothers should go through medical school... Well, for at least one year... That way there would not be so many kids going to the doctor for just a simple cough!"

—Miranda Connelly, 4th Grader

Alas, there is not a simple solution for such complex problem of low health literacy. It takes a village to raise a child, and it takes each and all parts involved in the process of effective health communication for improved health outcomes. Even the definition of health literacy is literally up for revision on the Roundtable on Health Literacy as of April of 2016, moving from individual skills in patients and providers, to systems and sources of health information in a multidimensional journey towards population health [15].

Health Literacy in Numbers

Prior to the publication of the 1992 National Adult Literacy (NAL) Survey, the extent of poor health literacy in the U.S. population was unknown [16, 17]. The NAL survey involved more than 26,000 adults and examined their knowledge of general literacy in three domains: prose, document, and quantitative. Approximately 21% of the population, between 40 and 44 million adults nationwide, demonstrated skills in the lowest level of proficiency, Level 1. Individuals functioning at this level are usually expected to read a relatively short text to locate a single piece of information, sign their name, find a country in a short article, and add a simple sum of numbers [16–18]. Individuals who function at this level are considered functionally illiterate. Another 27% of the population, representing as many as 54 million adults, demonstrated marginal literacy proficiency skills (Level 2). The surveyors also found that a gap exists between actual performance and self-evaluation of the interviewee's own skills. For example, of those adults who performed at Level 1 in prose literacy, only 34% said they did not write English well; 29% said they did not read English well.

A follow-up survey, the 2003 National Assessment of Adult Literacy (NAAL), reexamined the issue [19]. More than 19,000 adults older than the age of 16 years participated. The same three domains of literacy were measured. The scoring, however, was slightly different in that the survey scored four levels of literacy: Below Basic, Basic, Intermediate, and Proficient. Below Basic and Basic corresponded fairly well to the 1992 Levels 1 and 2. This was the first study to measure health literacy [20], and the data were published separately in September 2006. A total of 36% of the surveyed population, encompassing more than 78 million persons, scored in either the Below Basic or Basic level: 22% had Basic health literacy, and14% had Below Basic health literacy [21]. Older individuals, those foreign-born or born in the United States to families in which English is a second language, those who had less than a high school education, and those living below the poverty level had lower health literacy scores [20]. High percentages of adults with Below Basic or Basic health literacy received their information about health issues from radio and television rather than print media [20].

Health Literacy Tasks by Literacy Skills Levels.

Whereas approximately 30 million U.S. adults had Below Basic literacy skills based on the 2003 NAAL, only 12% scored Proficient health literacy skills (NCES 2006).

The following examples describe the literacy skills levels according to the health literacy tasks that individuals can do (NCES 2006):

1. *Below Basic*: individuals with the most simple and concrete literacy skills, who can follow instructions in simple forms, such as complete a social security card application
2. *Basic*: individuals who can perform simple and everyday literacy activities such as understand information in simple documents, locate quantitative information, and solve a one-step problem when an arithmetic operation is specified
3. *Intermediate*: individuals who can perform moderately challenging literacy activities such as read dense text, summarize, make inferences about the information; perform arithmetic operation not specified
4. *Proficient*: individuals who can perform more complex and challenging activities such as read and summarize complex information; perform multiple-step problems, arithmetic operation not specified

Below are examples of health literacy tasks, by level of complexity and literacy skill levels 8882 (NAAL 2006):

1. *Below Basic* (13%): can circle the appointment date and time on a hospital appointment slip; can follow a set of short instructions about what to do in preparation for a medical test
2. *Basic* (22%): can give two reasons why a person with no symptoms should have a test for the disease after reading information in a clearly written pamphlet
3. *Intermediate* (53%): can heed warnings about possible drug interactions based on over-the-counter medication labels; can determine when to take a pill 'on an empty stomach,' based on the medication label; can identify when a child needs a vaccine, based on vaccination schedules; can find the healthy weight range for a person in a body mass index chart
4. *Proficient* (12%): can find the information to explain a medical term by reading a complex document; can calculate the health insurance costs for a year with information from a table showing costs based on income and family size1

How Do We Know When a Patient Has Poor Literacy Skills?

The simple answer to the above question is, *"We don't."* In fact, clinicians frequently overestimate the literacy skills of patients and parents [22, 23]. Parikh et al., reported that 91% of individuals had not told their supervisor; 53% had not told their children; 68% had not told their spouse, and 19% had not told anyone about their poor literacy skills! [24]. Sometimes clues provided by the patient indicate difficulty with health literacy [18]. For instance, they may appear to be non-compliant: missing appointments, not taking their medications, failing to follow-through [18, 24, 25]. Cornett noted several other indications of probable poor literacy skills [26]:

- Patients often make excuses when asked to read (e.g., "I don't have my glasses" or "I'll read this when I get home.") or fill out forms, or they do not fill out forms completely.
- Poor readers point to the text with a finger while reading or lift the document close to their eyes, which seem to wander all over the page.
- Patients may check items as "no" on a medical history form to avoid having to answer follow-up questions.
- Individuals with poor health literacy identify pills by color, size, and/or shape, as they are not able to read the labels.
- Patients often show signs of nervousness, confusion, frustration, anger, or inappropriate happiness and even indifference. They may withdraw or avoid situations where complex learning is required.

Medication review is an excellent opportunity to identify health literacy issues. Patients with poor literacy skills will open a medicine bottle, take out a pill or look into the bottle and say "this is my yellow pill for blood pressure" because they cannot read the label. Individuals with poor literacy skills tend to be quite concrete in their reasoning and will have difficulties following abstract instructions such as 'take on an empty stomach'. They also may be unable to explain the timing for administration of a medication or explain a medication's purpose [18]. Reviewing the social history can be helpful to identify the extent of schooling completed. Of high school graduates, 15% scored in the Below Basic category, and 17% of NAAL participants who completed a college education had general literacy skills at the Basic or Below Basic levels [19]. Another way to get an idea of parents' literacy skills is to ask them if they read to their children or enjoy reading.

Measuring Health Literacy Skills

While it is appropriate to objectively measure patients' health literacy in a formal study about the impact of poor health literacy on health outcomes, some researchers have expressed concern that universal screening may not be helpful and may cause anxiety in individuals with very low health literacy skills [26]. Some of the health literacy screening tools will be briefly discussed in this section for those who are pursuing scholarly work [27].

Clinical screening, however, can negatively impact patient care by stigmatizing and labeling patients; Paasche-Orlow and Wolf found no evidence to support this routine practice [28].

Two tests are used primarily in the research setting, as they require a certain amount of time and skill to administer. These are the Test of Functional Health

Literacy in Adults (TOFHLA) and the Rapid Estimate of Adult Literacy in Medicine (REALM). Both of these tools were developed in the 1990s. TOFHLA is available in both English and Spanish and has a short form available. It also measures an individual's health literacy. The REALM estimates a patient's reading level and, because it uses medical terms, provides an estimate of health literacy. The REALM-R, a recent shorter version, takes only 2 min to administer, but it has not been validated as thoroughly as has the longer version.

A newer short test, the Newest Vital Sign (NVS), is a six-item assessment of a patient's ability to read and comprehend an ice cream nutrition label. This instrument can be accessed online free-of-charge and requires a maximum administration time of 6.2 min (average, 2.9 min). The correlation among the three tools is moderate.

Two other screening tools are the eHealth Literacy Scale (eHEALS), which tests perceived skills at finding and using electronic health information, and the Health Literacy Screening Question Methodologies (HLSQM), which identifies patients with inadequate health literacy but is not very efficient at identifying patients with marginal literacy abilities.

The Cost of Low Health Literacy and the Burden of Chronic Disease

"...interventions targeting parents likely to have low health literacy have an impact in reducing ED utilization." (p. 421)

—Morrison et al.

At least 80 million adults in the U.S. have poor health literacy skills [29], resulting in poor health choices, increased health costs, poor educational performance, and increased health disparities [18, 29, 30]. Low health literacy affects other groups such as the unemployed, low income, lack of a high school education [18]. Health and health care in the U.S. are increasingly characterized by technological sophistication. Thus, without adequate health literacy, this technological progress will exacerbate disparities over time [30].

Latinos have been identified as having lower levels of health literacy than other racial and ethnic groups in the U.S. [31]. Calvo recently examined a nationally representative sample of 2996 immigrants from the 2007 Pew Hispanic Center and Robert Wood Johnson Foundation Hispanic Healthcare Survey. Those individuals with higher levels of health literacy described better quality of care, regardless of health insurance coverage, degree of English proficiency, income, education, or having a medical home [31].

Low health literacy skills result in poor dietary habits, higher incidence of obesity [32, 33], higher rates of diabetes and metabolic syndrome [34]. Children with chronic conditions such as diabetes, must follow dietary recommendations to limit sugar and carbohydrates. Pulgarón and colleagues found that lower parental diabetes-related numeracy and lower perceived diabetes self-efficacy were inversely correlated to their children's glycemic control, regardless of their reading skills [35].

The link between low levels of health literacy and poor eating habits is very well illustrated by the work of Zoellner et al. [36]. They studied the healthy eating index (HEI) scores, as well as sugar-sweetened beverage intake in a group of adults with very low literacy scores—73.9% scored in the lowest two categories, Below Basic and Basic Literacy Skills. While controlling for all other variables, they found that HEI scores increased in a fixed relationship to increases in health literacy: each 1-point increase in health literacy equated to a 1.21-point increase in HEI scores. The intake of sugar-sweetened drinks was inversely related to health literacy; the higher the literacy level the less intake [36].

In the case of immunizations, the role that health literacy plays is not as clear. Ciampa and colleagues found no relationship between health literacy and lack of immunizations in their children, as did Pati [37, 38]. However, in the case of influenza vaccine, several studies have noted that older members of families with the poorest health literacy levels are less immunized, although this was not the case in the children [38, 39].

Parents with low health literacy skills are less compliant and less likely to follow medical recommendations for their children [40]. Mattar et al., reported that only 7.3% of parents where fully compliant with recommendations, while 53% of the children in the study took less than half of the medication [41]. Non-adherence is not a new phenomenon, however. In fact, it dates from at least the fourth century B.C.E. In his *Decorum*, Hippocrates states that one should "keep watch also on the fault of patients which often make them lie about the taking of things prescribed" [42].

The consequences of non-adherence are expensive and can be severe. In the U.S. the overall costs associated with non-adherence to medication regimens amount to $100 billion annually [43]. Hospitalization costs $13.35 billion [44]. Non-adherence to drug treatments also can have a significant impact on the prognosis of numerous disease states such as hypertension, diabetes, cancer. For example, pediatric patients with acute lymphocytic leukemia or Hodgkin disease who were non-adherent to their prednisone regimen had a 45% rate of relapse, significantly higher than the 10% of the adherent group [45]. In pediatric patients with renal transplants, non-adherence to immunosuppressive therapy leads to the need for more grafts, shorter graft survival, and increased mortality rates [46]. Parental low health literacy resulted in worse asthma control and poorer outcomes for children with asthma [47]. A systematic review of the literature by Morrison et al. found that parents with low health literacy skills used the emergency room more often for their children's asthma problems [48].

In summary, low health literacy results in higher health care costs and negative health outcomes for children, especially those with chronic conditions. Pediatric providers not only overestimate parental levels of health literacy [48], but they often forget that most patients do not understand medical jargon or *medicaleze*. Later on in this book we will expand on avoiding medical jargon—multi-syllable words, medical terminology, and compound sentences—as well as other strategies from the Health Literacy Universal Precaution Toolkit such as limiting amount of information given at a time, teach back and show me techniques for checking for understanding and using pictures and models.

Low Health Literacy and Patients' Experiences of Health Care

"Everybody gets so much information all day long that they lose their common sense"
—Gertrude Stein

Inadequate comprehension of medical information on the part of patients and parents is wide-spread. A recent study reported by Wynia and Osborn examined the results of a nationwide survey sent to 5929 adult patients by 13 healthcare organizations [49]. Health literacy obstacles were frequently reported. These included a lack of confidence in understanding written information, an inability to read without assistance information presented to them, and medical forms that were beyond comprehension. Additionally, individuals with low literacy skills use a variety of techniques to hide their low literacy and tend to limit their engagements in conversation for the same reason. This feeling of inadequacy can impair the patient's potential to benefit from health services and patient-professional communication as noted in the studies by Easton et al. and Smith et al. [50, 51]. In another study by Parikh and colleagues, almost 40% of patients with low functional literacy and poor reading ability admitted to having feelings of shame [52]. The stigma and shame associated with low literacy may lead to the depressive symptoms, as found by Smith and Moore in their study of low-literacy caregivers [24].

The difficulties that pediatric patients face as a result of their parents' or their own poor literacy and/or numeracy skills are not well studied, but parental low health literacy appears to impact the totality of health care for their children [53, 54]. A small study by Jimenez et al., examined understanding of the Early Intervention program by parents with low health literacy [53]. The parents reported that: "(1) they lacked continuity with a single pediatrician, (2) they had difficulty contacting the Early Intervention program, (3) they were confused about Early Intervention or the referral process (4) their pediatricians did not explain the Program and (5) written materials provided to them were not helpful" [53]. Kumar and colleagues noted that among parents with low literacy, only 47% could correctly describe how to mix infant formula from concentrate and 69% could interpret a digital thermometer [54]. A study of pediatric emergency department usage found that a median of 30% (interquartile range 22–36%) of parents in the emergency department possessed low health literacy [55], which is in keeping with national data [56].

Some data strongly suggest that low health literacy among adolescents negatively impacts their health experience. Children receiving Medicaid have levels of obesity higher than those of the general population, with 25.6% of 12- to 19-year-olds receiving Medicaid in Maryland being obese [57], compared to 20.8% of 14-year-old adolescents in the general population [58]. Chari et al., have shown that obesity in school-aged children is associated with parental factors including low health literacy, whereas obesity in adolescents is strongly associated with an adolescent's own low health literacy [32]. Sharif and Blank reported similar findings in a cohort of overweight children: low literacy negatively correlated with the degree of obesity ($r = -0.37$, $p = 0.0009$) [33].

What about pediatric patients with specific medical conditions? Pediatric patients with asthma who utilize emergency departments are also ill-served if their parents have poor literacy skills [59, 60]. For example, Deise and colleagues found that poor literacy skills were associated with inadequate knowledge about daily administration of an inhaled corticosteroid [59]. Macy and co-workers found that the health literacy levels were low in 31% of the parents seen in an emergency department setting and that high scores on knowledge of asthma at enrollment to their study were achieved by only 33% of low-literacy parents, compared to 59% of adequate-health-literacy parents (p = 0.025) [60]. Gandhi et al., examined the relationships among health literacy, self-efficacy with patient physician interactions, and asthma control. They reported that parents with higher health literacy and greater perceived self-efficacy were associated with higher satisfaction with shared decision-making. Further, greater satisfaction with shared decision-making was associated with better asthma control [61]. Conversely, low parental health literacy has been associated with poor measures of care in children with asthma [62]. Children of parents with low literacy had greater incidences of emergency department visits, hospitalizations, and days missed from school. They also used rescue medications more often.

The management of the other prevalent pediatric chronic disease, diabetes, is strongly influenced by parental health literacy and parental education. In adults, a direct relationship exists among health numeracy, health literacy, and greater diabetes self-efficacy, with greater diabetes self-efficacy being associated with better glycemic control [63]. Pulgarón and colleagues demonstrated that parental diabetes-related numeracy (health literacy) and perceived diabetes self-efficacy, but not reading skills, per se, were inversely correlated with the child's glycemic control [35].

Parents with low health literacy used non-standard dosing tools more often and this can lead to medication errors [64–66]. Yin et al., in particular, noted that inadequate or marginal overall health literacy was linked with a lack of knowledge of weight-based dosing [65]. Medication errors associated with poor recall of instructions for administration appears to be true for all literacy levels [67]. Adherence to a long-term medication regimen may also be adversely impacted by poor health literacy on the part of the parents [68]. Chapter 3 will address in detail the relationship between low health literacy and medication errors.

Adolescents transitioning from pediatric to adult care are another major population for which a lack of literacy skills can adversely affect the continuity of care. Transition is difficult at best, but it is further complicated if the adolescent has poor health literacy skills [69–71]. Clinicians frequently overestimate the adolescent patient's literacy skills, as well as those of their parents, when judging the health literacy-related readiness for transition to adult care of pediatric patients [22, 23, 71].

References

1. Definition of "Communication" Merriam-Webseter.com. Merriam-Webster; n.d. Web. http://www.merriam-webster.com/dictionary/communication. Accessed 11 May 2016.
2. Griffith CH, Wilson JF, Langer S, Haist SA. House staff nonverbal communication skills and standardized patient satisfaction. J Gen Intern Med. 2003;18(3):170–4. doi:10.1046/j.1525-1497.2003.10506.

3. Ha JF, Longnecker N. Doctor-patient communication: a review. Ochsner J. 2010;10(1):38–43.
4. Teutsch C. Patient-doctor communication. Med Clin North Am. 2003;87(5):1115–45.5.
5. Schyve PM. Language differences as a barrier to quality and safety in health care: the Joint Commission perspective. J Gen Intern Med. 2007;22(Suppl 2):360–1. doi:10.1007/s11606-007-0365-3.
6. U.S. Department of Health and Human Services, Office of Disease Prevention and Health Promotion. National action plan to improve health literacy. Washington: Author; 2010.
7. Quote from Rear Admiral Kenneth P. Moritsugu, MD, MPH—Acting United States Surgeon General, found in the Centers for Disease Control and Prevention Lead Health Literacy Initiative Web. http://www.cdc.gov/nceh/lead/tools/leadliteracy.htm. Accessed 11 May 2016.
8. Definition of "Literacy" Merriam-Webseter.com. Merriam-Webster; n.d. Web. http://www.merriam-webster.com/dictionary/literacy. Accessed 11 May 2016.
9. National Assessment of Adult Literacy Definition of Literacy. https://nces.ed.gov/naal/fr_definition.asp. Accessed 11 May 2016.
10. "What is Health Literacy?" Report brief health literacy: a prescription to end confusion. National Academies Press Web. http://www.nationalacademies.org/hmd/~/media/Files/Report%20Files/2004/Health-Literacy-A-Prescription-to-End-Confusion/healthliteracyfinal.pdf. Accessed 11 May 2016.
11. Institute of Medicine (US) Roundtable on Health Literacy. Measures of health literacy: workshop summary. Washington: National Academies Press; 2009. 6, Measuring health literacy: what? So what? Now what? http://wwwncbinlmnihgov/books/NBK45386/. Accessed 1 June 2016.
12. Definition of "Universal Precautions" United States Department of Labor Occupational Safety and Health Administration OSHA Web. https://www.osha.gov/SLTC/etools/hospital/hazards/univprec/univ.html. Accessed 1 June 2016.
13. What are health literacy universal precautions? Agency for Healthcare Research and Quality AHRQ Web. http://www.ahrq.gov/professionals/quality-patient-safety/quality-resources/tools/literacy-toolkit/index.html. Accessed 1 June 2016.
14. Definition of "Common Sense" Merriam-Webster.com. Merriam-Webster; n.d. Web. http://www.merriam-webster.com/dictionary/common%20sense. Accessed 11 May 2016.
15. Pleasant A, Rudd RE, O'Leary C, Paasche-Orlow MK, Allen MP, Alvarado-Little W, Myers L, Parson K, Rosen S. Considerations for a new definition of health literacy. Discussion paper. Washington: National Academy of Medicine. http://nam.edu/wp-content/uploads/2016/04/Considerations-for-a-New-Definition-ofHealth-Literacy.pdf. Accessed 1 June 2016.
16. Kirsch I, Jungeblut A, Jenkins L, et al. Adult literacy in America: a first look at the results of the National Adult Literacy Survey. Washington: National Center for Education Statistics, US Department of Education; 1993.
17. https://nces.ed.gov/pubs93/93275.pdf. Accessed 5 Feb 2016.
18. Weiss BD. Health literacy: a manual for clinicians. Chicago: American Medical Association Foundation and American Medical Association; 2003.
19. http://files.eric.ed.gov/fulltext/ED493284.pdf. Accessed Feb 2016.
20. http://nces.ed.gov/pubs2006/2006483.pdf. Accessed 5 Feb 2016.
21. http://datacenter.kidscount.org/data/tables/99-total-population-by-child-and-adult#detailed/1/any/false/869,36,868,867,14/39,40,41/416,417. Accessed 5 Feb 2016.
22. Bass III PF, Wilson JF, Griffith CH, et al. Residents' ability to identify patients with poor literacy skills. Acad Med. 2002;77(10):1039–41.
23. Kelly PA, Haidet P. Physician overestimation of patient literacy: a potential source of health care disparities. Patient Educ Couns 2007;66(1):119–22.
24. Parikh NS, Parker RM, Nurss JR, et al. Shame and health literacy: the unspoken connection. Patient Educ Couns. 1996;27(1):33–9.
25. Baker DW, Parker RM, Williams MV, et al. The health care experience of patients with low literacy. Arch Fam Med. 1996;5(6):329–34.
26. Cornett S. Assessing and addressing health literacy. Online J of Issues in Nursing 2009;14. http://www.nursingworld.org/MainMenuCategories/ANAMarketplace/ANAPeriodicals/

OJIN/TableofContents/Vol142009/No3Sept09/Assessing-Health-Literacy-.html. Accessed 5 Feb 2016.

27. Collins SA, Currie LM, Bakken S, et al. Health literacy screening instruments for eHealth applications: a systematic review. J Biomed Inform. 2012;45(3):598–607.

28. Paasche-Orlow MK, Wolf MS. Evidence does not support clinical screening of literacy. J Gen Intern Med. 2008;23(1):100–2.

29. http://nces.ed.gov/pubs2006/2006483.pdf. Accessed 10 Feb 2016.

30. Parker RM, Ratzan SC, Lurie N. Health literacy: a policy challenge for advancing high-quality health care. Health Aff. 2003;22(4):147–53.

31. Calvo R. Health literacy and quality of care among Latino immigrants in the United States. Health Soc Work. 2016;41(1):e44–51.

32. Chari R, Warsh J, Ketterer T, et al. Association between health literacy and child and adolescent obesity. Patient Educ Couns. 2014;94(1):61–6.

33. Sharif I, Blank AE. Relationship between child health literacy and body mass index in overweight children. Patient Educ Couns. 2010;79(1):43–8.

34. https://www.idf.org/metabolic-syndrome/children. Accessed 12 Feb 2016.

35. Pulgarón ER, Sanders LM, Patiño-Fernandez AM, et al. Glycemic control in young children with diabetes: the role of parental health literacy. Patient Educ Couns. 2014;94(1):67–70.

36. Zoellner J, You W, Connel C, et al. Health literacy is associated with healthy eating index scores and sugar-sweetened beverage intake: findings from the rural Lower Mississippi Delta. J Am Diet Assoc. 2011;111(7):1012–20.

37. Ciampa PJ, White RO, Perrin EM, et al. The association of acculturation and health literacy, numeracy and health-related skills in Spanish-speaking caregivers of young children. J Immigr Minor Health. 2013;15(3):492–8.

38. Pati S, Feemster KA, Mohamad Z, et al. Maternal health literacy and late initiation of immunizations among an inner-city birth cohort. Matern Child Health J. 2011;15(3):386–94.

39. Berkman ND, Sheridan SL, Donahue KE, et al. Health literacy interventions and outcomes: an updated systematic review. Evidence Report/Technology Assessment No. 199. Prepared by RTI International–University of North Carolina Evidence based Practice Center under contract No. 290-2007-10056-I. AHRQ Publication Number 11-E006. Rockville: Agency for Healthcare Research and Quality; 2011.

40. Fotheringham MJ, Sawyer MG. Adherence to recommended medical regimens in childhood and adolescence. J Paediatr Child Health. 1995;31:72–8.

41. Mattar ME, Markello J, Yaffe SJ. Inadequacies in the pharmacologic management of ambulatory children. J Pediatr. 1975;87:137–41.

42. Carrick P. Medical ethics in the ancient world. Washington: Georgetown University Press; 2001. p 105.

43. Osterberg L, Blaschke T. Adherence to medication. N Engl J Med. 2005;353:487–97.

44. Martin LR, Williams SL, Haskard KB, et al. The challenge of patient adherence. Ther Clin Risk Manag. 2005;1:189–99.

45. Festa RS, Tamaroff MH, Chasalow F, et al. Therapeutic adherence to oral medication regimens by adolescents with cancer. I. Laboratory assessment. J Pediatr. 1991;120:807–11.

46. Meyers KE, Weiland H, Thomson PD. Paediatric renal transplantation non-compliance. Pediatr Nephrol. 1995;9:189–92.

47. Harrington KF, Zhang B, Magruder T, Bailey WC, Gerald LB. The impact of parent's health literacy on pediatric asthma outcomes. Pediatr Allergy Immunol Pulmonol. 2015;28(1):20–6. doi:10.1089/ped.2014.0379.

48. Morrisonon AK, Myrvik MP, Brousseau DC, Hoffmann RG, Stanley RM. The relationship between parent health literacy and pediatric emergency department utilization: a systematic review. Acad Pediatr. 2013;13(5):421–9. doi:10.1016/j.acap.2013.03.001.

49. Wynia MK, Osborn CY. Health literacy and communication quality in health care organizations. J Health Commun. 2010;15(Suppl 2):102–15.

50. Easton P, Entwistle VA, Williams B. How the stigma of low literacy can impair patient-professional spoken interactions and affect health: insights from a qualitative investigation. BMC Health Serv Res. 2013;13:319.

51. Smith SG, Wolf MS, von Wagner C. Socioeconomic status, statistical confidence, and patient-provider communication: an analysis of the Health Information National Trends Survey (HINTS 2007). J Health Commun. 2010;15(Suppl 3):169–85.
52. Smith SA, Moore EJ. Health literacy and depression in the context of home visitation. Matern Child Health J. 2012;16(7):1500–8.
53. Jimenez ME, Barg FK, Guevara JP, et al. The impact of parental health literacy on the early intervention referral process. J Health Care Poor Underserved. 2013;24(3):1053–62.
54. Kumar D, Sanders L, Perrin EM, et al. Parental understanding of infant health information: health literacy, numeracy, and the Parental Health Literacy Activities Test (PHLAT). Acad Pediatr. 2010;10(5):309–16.
55. Morrisonon AK, Myrvik MP, Brousseau DC, et al. The relationship between parent health literacy and pediatric emergency department utilization: a systematic review. Acad Pediatr. 2013;13(5):421–9.
56. Paasche-Orlow MK, Parker RM, Gazmararian JA, et al. The prevalence of limited health literacy. J Gen Intern Med. 2005;20(2):175–84.
57. Hurt L, Pinto CD, Watson J, et al; Centers for Disease Control and Prevention (CDC). Diagnosis and screening for obesity-related conditions among children and teens receiving Medicaid—Maryland, 2005-2010. MMWR Morb Mortal Wkly Rep. 2014;63(14):305–8.
58. Cunningham SA, Kramer MR, Narayan KMV. Incidence of childhood obesity in the United States. N Engl J Med. 2014;370:403–11.
59. Deis JN, Spiro DM, Jenkins CA, et al. Parental knowledge and use of preventive asthma care measures in two pediatric emergency departments. J Asthma. 2010 Jun;47(5):551–6.
60. Macy ML, Davis MM, Clark SJ, et al. Parental health literacy and asthma education delivery during a visit to a community-based pediatric emergency department: a pilot study. Pediatr Emerg Care. 2011;27(6):469–74.
61. Gandhi PK, Kenzik KM, Thompson LA, et al. Exploring factors influencing asthma control and asthma-specific health-related quality of life among children. Respir Res. 2013;14:26.
62. DeWalt D, Dilling N, Rosenthal M, Pignone M. Low parental literacy is associated with worse asthma care measures in children. Ambul Pediatr. 2007;7:25–31.
63. Osborn CY, Cavanaugh K, Wallston KA, et al. Self-efficacy links health literacy and numeracy to glycemic control. J Health Commun. 2010;15(Suppl 2):146–58.
64. Tanner S, Wells M, Scarbecz M, et al. Parents' understanding of and accuracy in using measuring devices to administer liquid oral pain medication. J Am Dent Assoc. 2014;145(2):141–9.
65. Yin HS, Dreyer BP, Foltin G, et al. Association of low caregiver health literacy with reported use of non-standardized dosing instruments and lack of knowledge of weight-based dosing. Ambul Pediatr. 2007;7(4):292–8.
66. Yin HS, Mendelsohn AL, Wolf MS, et al. Parents' medication administration errors: role of dosing instruments and health literacy. Arch Pediatr Adolesc Med. 2010;164:181–6.
67. Bayldon BW, Glusman M, Fortuna NM, et al. Exploring caregiver understanding of medications immediately after a pediatric primary care visit. Patient Educ Couns. 2013;91(2):255–60.
68. Freedman RB, Jones SK, Lin A, et al. Influence of parental health literacy and dosing responsibility on pediatric glaucoma medication adherence. Arch Ophthalmol. 2012;130(3):306–11.
69. Ferris ME, Cuttance JR, Javalkar K, et al. Self-management and transition among adolescents/young adults with chronic or end-stage kidney disease. Blood Purif. 2015;39(1–3):99–104.
70. Lewis SA, Noyes J. Effective process or dangerous precipice: qualitative comparative embedded case study with young people with epilepsy and their parents during transition from children's to adult services. BMC Pediatr. 2013 Oct;13:169.
71. Huang JS, Tobin A, Tompanc T. Clinicians poorly assess health literacy-related readiness for transition to adult care in adolescents with inflammatory bowel disease. Clin Gastroenterol Hepatol. 2012;10(6):626–32.

Chapter 2
Health Literacy and Child Health Outcomes: From Prenatal to Birth and Infant Stages

Michael E. Speer

The impact of parental health literacy and the health outcomes of young children is a poorly studied area. DeWalt et al., summarized the pertinent literature regarding literacy and child outcomes, not necessarily health literacy, from 1980 through 2008 [1]. They presented 24 studies that dealt with the relationship between literacy and child health outcomes and found that lower literacy was associated with a lack of basic knowledge regarding a known medical condition, difficulty utilizing consent forms, non-comprehension of the concepts behind prenatal screening, and non-understanding of educational brochures resulting in poorer health outcomes.

However, the impact of health literacy on a baby occurs before birth or even before pregnancy [1]. Gossett and co-workers demonstrated that lower health literacy is associated with limited appreciation of the implications of aging on fertility and pregnancy, and the success rates of infertility treatments [2].

Low literacy and numeracy scores are also associated with poor knowledge about contraception and difficulty with use of contraceptives [3]. Individuals with low health literacy skills are less likely to use the Internet and more likely to have self-efficacy limitations [4]. Thus, a program such as Text4baby, which has "a free cell phone text messaging service for pregnant women and new moms" and provides "text messages [that] are sent three times a week with information on how to have a healthy pregnancy and a healthy baby" [5] succeeds best with individuals with higher health literacy levels [6, 7]. In studies of pregestational diabetics [8] and gestational diabetics [9], those with poor health literacy had significantly more unplanned pregnancies, had not discussed pregnancy planning with a physician, or had taken folic acid. Their literacy level had a significant

M.E. Speer, M.D. (✉)
Professor of Pediatrics and Ethics, Section of Neonatology, Department of Pediatrics, Baylor College of Medicine, Texas Children's Hospital, Houston, TX, USA

© The Editor(s) and The Author(s) 2017   15
R.A. Connelly, T. Turner (eds.), *Health Literacy and Child Health Outcomes*,
SpringerBriefs in Public Health, DOI 10.1007/978-3-319-50799-6_2

impact regarding their understanding of information about gestational diabetes mellitus [9]. Similar findings were found by You and colleagues with regard to knowledge about preeclampsia [10]. As both diabetes and pre-eclampsia are associated with preterm birth [11, 12, 13], there is an increased risk of lung disease, infection, and other complications that adversely impact health outcomes throughout life. Interestingly, the level of health literacy does not seem to predict smoking during pregnancy [14].

Low parental literacy affects almost every aspect of newborn and infant care, including breastfeeding, use of the emergency room, medication administration, and participation in social welfare programs. Kaufman and co-workers found that only 23% of first-time mothers with poor health literacy breast-fed exclusively for 2 months, compared to 54% of women who had higher levels of literacy skills [15].

With regard to the emergency room environment, Morrison and colleagues reported that as many as two thirds of caregivers presenting with their children had low health literacy, and these individuals had more than three times greater odds of presenting to the emergency center for a non-urgent conditions than did those with adequate health literacy. They also found that health literacy was an independent predictor of higher use of the emergency room for non-urgent conditions [16, 17].

Problems involving administration of medication, including the use of non-standard measuring devices, are well known when caregivers have low literacy [18–20]. Caregivers with lower numeracy skills were also more likely to provide inappropriate reasons for giving an over-the-counter medication [21]. Wallace et al., found that both directions for preparation and instructions for the use and storage of powdered infant formulas' labels had average reading scores at the college level. The Warnings and Safe Handling sections had reading difficulty levels between the 8th- and 9th-grade levels, inviting misinterpretation of proper formula preparation [22].

Participation in social programs such as Temporary Assistance for Needy Families (TANF), the Food Stamp Program, and Special Supplemental Nutrition Program for Women, Infants, and Children (WIC) are critical to healthy nutrition and normal development. Pati et al., found that participation in TANF was more than twice as common among children whose mothers had adequate health literacy compared with children whose mothers had inadequate health literacy [23]. Low health literacy also may contribute to gaps in Medicaid coverage, particularly when the caregivers have less than a high school education [24].

Lack of up-to-date immunizations at either age 3 or 7 months was related to education level (high school graduate or beyond), attending a hospital-affiliated clinic [25], and maternal employment [26], but not to the level of health literacy [25].

A problem with many studies on the impact of health literacy on children's health is that they rely on reported parental behavior, rather than measured behavior [27]. Unfortunately, self-reported data about participation are subject to recall bias and, depending on response rates, selection bias [23]. Thus, appropriately designed studies on this topic are critical to (1) accurately measure the impact of health literacy on caregivers' actions separate from other known influences and (2) hopefully narrow the gap between children's health outcomes seen in high- versus low-literacy caregivers.

References

1. DeWalt DA, Hink A. Health literacy and child health outcomes: A systematic review of the literature. Pediatrics. 2009;124(3 suppl):S265–74.
2. Gossett DR, Nayak S, Bhatt S, Bailey SC. What do healthy women know about the consequences of delayed childbearing? J Health Commun. 2013;18(1 Suppl):118–28.
3. Yee LM, Simon MA. The role of health literacy and numeracy in contraceptive decision-making for urban Chicago women. J Community Health. 2014;39(2):394–9.
4. Shieh C, Mays R, McDaniel A, Yu J. Health literacy and its association with the use of information sources and with barriers to information seeking in clinic-based pregnant women. Health Care Women Int. 2009;30(11):971–88.
5. Text4baby. http://www.cdc.gov/women/text4baby/. Accessed 19 Jan 2016.
6. Gazmararian JA, Elon L, Yang B, et al. Text4baby program: an opportunity to reach underserved pregnant and postpartum women? Matern Child Health J. 2014;18(1):223–32.
7. Gazmararian JA, Yang B, Elon L, et al. Successful enrollment in Text4Baby more likely with higher health literacy. J Health Commun. 2012;17(3 Suppl):303–11.
8. Endres LK, Sharp LK, Haney E, Dooley SL. Health literacy and pregnancy preparedness in pregestational diabetes. Diabetes Care. 2004;27(2):331–4.
9. Carolan M. Diabetes nurse educators' experiences of providing care for women, with gestational diabetes mellitus, from disadvantaged backgrounds. J Clin Nurs. 2014;23(9–10):1374–84.
10. You WB, Wolf MS, Bailey SC, et al. Improving patient understanding of preeclampsia: a randomized controlled trial. Am J Obstet Gynecol. 2012;206(5):431.e1–5.
11. Köck K, Köck F, Klein K, et al. Diabetes mellitus and the risk of preterm birth with regard to the risk of spontaneous preterm birth. J Matern Fetal Neonatal Med. 2010;23(9):1004–8.
12. Preeclampsia. http://www.marchofdimes.org/complications/preeclampsia.aspx. Accessed 19 Jan 2016
13. Xaverius P, Alman C, Holtz L, et al. Risk factors associated with very low birth weight in a large urban area, stratified by adequacy of prenatal care. Matern Child Health J. 2015;4. [Epub ahead of print]
14. Arnold CL, Davis TC, Berkel HJ, et al. Smoking status, reading level, and knowledge of tobacco effects among low-income pregnant women. Prev Med. 2001;32(4):313–20.
15. Kaufman H, Skipper B, Small L, et al. Effect of literacy on breast-feeding outcomes. South Med J. 2001;94(3):293–6.
16. Morrison AK, Schapira MM, Gorelick MH, et al. Low caregiver health literacy is associated with higher pediatric emergency department use and nonurgent visits. Acad Pediatr. 2014;14(3):309–14.
17. Morrison AK, Chanmugathas R, Schapira MM, et al. Caregiver low health literacy and nonurgent use of the pediatric emergency department for febrile illness. Acad Pediatr. 2014;14(5):505–9.
18. Yin HS, Dreyer BP, Foltin G, et al. Association of low caregiver health literacy with reported use of nonstandardized dosing instruments and lack of knowledge of weight-based dosing. Ambul Pediatr. 2007;7(4):292–8.
19. Mira JJ, Lorenzo S, Guilabert M, et al. A systematic review of patient medication error on self-administering medication at home. Expert Opin Drug Saf. 2015;14(6):815–38.
20. Mehndiratta S. Strategies to reduce medication errors in pediatric ambulatory settings. J Postgrad Med. 2012;58(1):47–53.
21. Lokker N, Sanders L, Perrin EM, et al. Parental misinterpretations of over-the-counter pediatric cough and cold medication labels. Pediatrics. 2009;123(6):1464–71.
22. Wallace LS, Rosenstein PF, Gal N. Readability and content characteristics of powdered infant formula instructions in the United States. Matern Child Health J. 2016;20(4):889–94. [Epub ahead of print]
23. Pati S, Mohamad Z, Cnaan A, et al. Influence of maternal health literacy on child participation in social welfare programs: the Philadelphia experience. Am J Public Health. 2010;100(9):1662–5.

24. Lee JY, Divaris K, DeWalt DA, et al. Caregivers' health literacy and gaps in children's Medicaid enrollment: findings from the Carolina Oral Health Literacy Study. PLoS One. 2014;9(10):e110178.
25. Pati S, Feemster KA, Mohamad Z, et al. Maternal health literacy and late initiation of immunizations among an inner-city birth cohort. Matern Child Health J. 2011;15(3):386–94.
26. Brenner RA, Simons-Morton BG, Bhaskar B, et al.; NIH-D.C. Initiative Immunization Group. Prevalence and predictors of immunization among inner-city infants: a birth cohort study. Pediatrics. 2001;108(3):661–70.
27. Knapp C, Madden V, Wang H. Internet use and eHealth literacy of low-income parents whose children have special health care needs. J Med Internet Res. 2011;13(3):e75.

Chapter 3
Health Literacy and Child Health Outcomes: Parental Health Literacy and Medication Errors

H. Shonna Yin

Medication Errors and Children

Parents frequently take on the task of dosing medications for their children. More than half of children in the US take one or more medications in a given week [1]. Unfortunately, every 8 min, a child experiences an outpatient medication error, and this estimate is based only on those errors that lead to U.S. Poison Control Center calls [2]. Parental medication administration errors are thought to account for 70% of preventable pediatric outpatient adverse events [3, 4].

Errors with medications range in type and can include quantitative dosing errors, in which a different amount is given than was intended, errors in frequency or duration, administration of an incorrect medication or formulation, use of an incorrect administration route, or incorrect preparation or storage [5–9].

Why are medication errors so frequent? It is likely that health literacy plays an important role. Numerous studies have linked low parent health literacy to medication errors [10–13]. In thinking about the construct of health literacy being at the intersection of an individual's abilities and the demands and complexities placed on individuals from the health care system, it is not unexpected that errors occur.

In pediatrics, the task of administering medications correctly can be complex. For children, especially young ones, providers typically rely on liquid formulations, as children may have difficulty swallowing pill form medicines. Dosing with liquid medications is confusing; in fact, over 80% of pediatric medication errors involve liquid formulations [2]. Studies have found that more than half of parents make

H. Shonna Yin, MD, MS (✉)
Associate Professor of Pediatrics and Population Health, Departments of Pediatrics and Population Health, NYU School of Medicine/Bellevue Hospital Center, 550 First Avenue, NBV 8S4-11, New York, NY 10016, USA
e-mail: yinh2@med.nyu.edu

© The Editor(s) and The Author(s) 2017
R.A. Connelly, T. Turner (eds.), *Health Literacy and Child Health Outcomes*, SpringerBriefs in Public Health, DOI 10.1007/978-3-319-50799-6_3

errors dosing liquid medications [14–18], and about 50% of pediatric caregivers do not adhere to their prescribed medication regimens [19, 20].

Medication errors result in emergency department visits and/or significant morbidity. The drug classes most commonly implicated include analgesics (opioids and non-opioids), antibiotics, central nervous system medications (anticonvulsants, antipsychotics, antidepressants, stimulants), cardiovascular drugs (e.g. clonidine), and gastrointestinal medications (e.g. metoclopramide) [6, 7, 21].

Health Literacy Challenge #1: Dosing Tools

One health literacy challenge with liquid medications is that parents must understand the importance of measurement tools and how to appropriately use them. A wide array of dosing tools can be used to measure medications (see Fig. 3.1). It has long been recognized that nonstandard kitchen spoons are inaccurate: an American Academy of Pediatrics (AAP) Policy Statement from 1975—over 40 years ago—recommended the use of standard dosing tools [22].

A recent Federal Drug Administration (FDA) guidance recommends inclusion of a standardized dosing tool with all over-the-counter liquid medicines [23]. Use of kitchen spoons has been found to be associated with over 2.5 times the odds of a medication error compared to when standardized tools are used [12, 24, 25].

Standardized tools, which include oral syringes, dosing spoons, dosing cups, and droppers, have markings which guide parents in the correct measurement of medicines. Kitchen spoons, on the other hand, vary widely in size and shape, making it difficult to measure the correct amount, contributing to over- and under-dosing [26].

While oral syringes have traditionally been considered the tool to use when accuracy is important in clinical settings, such as hospitals and pharmacies, there is no existing national guidance regarding which dosing tool to provide when prescription

Fig. 3.1 Some of the wide arrays of tools parents use to measure liquid medications. *Photo by H. Shonna Yinn*

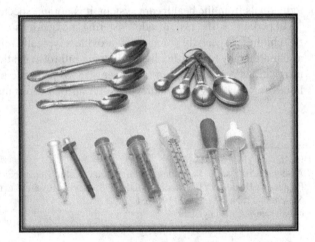

medications are dispensed [16, 19, 27]. And while dosing cups are the most common dosing tools included with over-the-counter medication packaging [28], several studies have documented that parents struggle to dose accurately using dosing cups, increasing the risk for overdose and multi-fold errors [11, 29].

Challenges in dosing accurately with cups include confusion that the full cup is the dose, or that each cup is one measurement unit, and not holding the cup at eye level when measuring the medication [11, 25]. New research is in progress examining implications of dosing tool type based on dose amounts, which suggest that the optimal tool used to measure a medication may vary based on the dose amount recommended [30].

Health Literacy Challenge #2: Units of Measurement

Another health literacy challenge related to appropriate parent administration of liquid medications is the lack of consistency in the language used as part of dosing instructions and accompanying dosing tools to describe units of measurement. Different terms may be used to describe dose amounts, including milliliter (mL), teaspoon (tsp), and tablespoon (TBSP); sometimes a milligram equivalent dose is provided [28, 31]. In rare cases, terms like cubic centimeter (cc) or drams may be seen [28]. Confusion between terms can result in multi-fold errors—either ineffective treatment with under-dosing or over-doses leading to toxic levels.

Example of Suboptimal Use of Units on Labeled Instructions and Dosing Tool, Resulting in Parent Confusion

A father bought diphenhydramine which came with a dosage cup that was prominently marked with a "12.5 mL" dose. The medication label indicated the correct dosage for his 5-year-old child was "12.5 mg–25 mg". The father subsequently poured 12.5 mL, not mg, of medication, which is the equivalent of 31.25 mg. Luckily, he caught his mistake before administering the medication to his child [32].

Example of mg Equivalent on Dosing Tool Leading to Confusion

A 6 year old child was prescribed oseltamivir following a diagnosis of H1N1 influenza. While the prescribed dose shown on the bottle label was specified with a volume of ¾ teaspoonful, the accompanying prepackaged syringe only had markings in milliliters. The correct dose was eventually calculated using information found in part of the package insert that was intended for prescribers, not parents [31].

Fig. 3.2 Inconsistencies
within same medication
label '**2 MILLILITERS**'
for instructions and '250
MG/**5 ML**' next to
medication name at the
bottom. *Photo by Rosina
Avila Connelly*

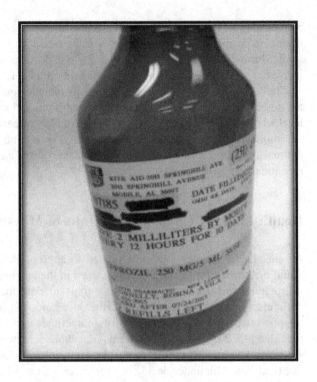

The use of units of measurement in over-the-counter (OTC) medications has been inconsistent. A study of 200 top-selling OTC liquid medications found that the majority of labels and associated dosing tools were not consistent in the use of units of measurement [28]. For example, a liquid medication for children had a dosing chart that recommended a dose of "2 teaspoons", but only a "2 TBS" measuring cup—2 tablespoon dose—was included in the package, increasing the likelihood of a threefold error [28].

Inconsistency is common with prescription medications as well. A study which compared units used on prescription labels with the units which were included on the medication bottle found that over a third had been altered—for example, one unit was switched for another, or another unit of measure was added [33]. This lack of consistency is likely to breed confusion (Fig. 3.2).

Concerns regarding the lack of standardization of units and resultant inconsistencies in labeling have led the Centers for Disease Control, through its PROTECT Initiative, to push for a move to mL-only dosing as well as elimination of teaspoon and tablespoon terms [34]. The AAP, which was a part of the PROTECT initiative, issued a Policy Statement supporting mL-only dosing in 2015 [35]. Other groups, including the American Academy of Family Practitioners (AAFP), American Association of Poison Control Center (AAPCC), and the Institute for Safe Medication Practices (ISMP), have been key partners in the PROTECT initiative and have come out in support of a move to mL-only dosing as well [36–38]. The benefit of a move to a single consistent unit is multifold—reducing confusion not only for parents, but also among health care providers. Cases have been reported of physicians mixing up units in calculating the amount of medication to be prescribed, as well as pharmacists mixing up units, resulting in errors in the dosing instructions when medications are dispensed.

The following cases illustrate the need for systems-based solutions which are likely to reduce medication errors.

Example of Confusion with Units Resulting in Error at the Point of Dispensing

A pharmacy label for a ranitidine prescription to treat gastroesophageal reflux disease was incorrectly dispensed to read "0.5 teaspoonful three times daily" instead of 0.5 mL three times daily, a fivefold error. The 8-month-old child developed tremors, excessive blinking, and trouble sleeping over the 2 weeks that the overdose was administered [39].

Example of Confusion with Units Resulting in Error at the Point of Dispensing

A pharmacist filling a prescription for daily 2.5 mL of azithromycin erroneously labeled the bottle with a dosage of 2.5 teaspoonfuls' daily, a 5-fold error. The medication was administered at the erroneous dose by the parent, whose child subsequently developed diarrhea [39].

Example of Confusion with Units Resulting in Error at the Point of Dispensing

A child who was discharged after surgery presented to the ED with respiratory distress. It was discovered that the child was given a prescription of Tylenol #3 (acetaminophen and codeine) but the label read six teaspoonful's every 4 h, and not the correct 6 mL. The child was admitted for his respiratory distress [40].

In addition, terms like teaspoon or tablespoon inadvertently endorse the use of nonstandard dosing tools. A recent study found that when "teaspoon" or "tsp" was included in dosing instructions, parents had a greater than four times increased odds of choosing a nonstandard tool, compared to when instructions were in mL only [30].

Health Literacy Challenge #3: Range of Recommended Dose Amounts, Different Liquid Concentrations

Yet another health literacy challenge is that the amount of medicine that a child should be given can range from less than 1 mL to over 30 mL. Medications for children are dosed based on weight, and medications come in varying strengths and concentrations, resulting in a range of possible doses.

Dosing instructions often involve amounts that may not be familiar for parents. In the US, which has traditionally relied on a non-metric system, the most common amounts are based on teaspoon equivalents—5, 7.5, 10, 12.5, 15 mL—however, it is not uncommon to see dose amounts outside of teaspoon equivalents [41].

Dose amounts may use whole numbers (5 mL expressed as 1 teaspoon) or involve fractions of a whole (7.5 mL expressed as 1- ½ teaspoons), and may even involve doses so specific that the recommended amount is several digits to the right of the decimal point. Liquid medication dosing is unlike dosing for pill-form medicines, where there are typically whole number doses, or occasionally half dose increments. For example, the oral syringe for infant ibuprofen lists doses of 0.625, 1.25, 1.875 mL which would be difficult to measure with a regular 5 mL oral syringe (see excerpt from HELPix below) [86].

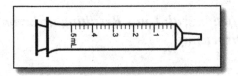

Decimal confusion can increase the risk of 10-fold errors, particularly when there is a lack of a leading zero (eg. "0.5 mL" confused for "5 mL") or when lagging zeroes are present ("1.0 mL" confused for "10 mL"). Such confusion has led to Joint Commission standard in the inpatient setting, but regulations which apply to the outpatient setting are lacking [42].

Health Literacy Challenges with Prescription Medications

A 5-year-old boy was discharged from the emergency department with a diagnosis of a viral syndrome and was prescribed liquid acetaminophen. Two days after discharge, the boy returned to ED, now complaining of fever, rigors, vomiting, lethargy, and right upper quadrant abdominal pain, with elevated acetaminophen levels. It was discovered that the parents misread instructions about dosing the prescribed liquid acetaminophen, giving 20 mL doses instead of 6 mL doses. The boy had to be admitted to the hospital for treatment [43].

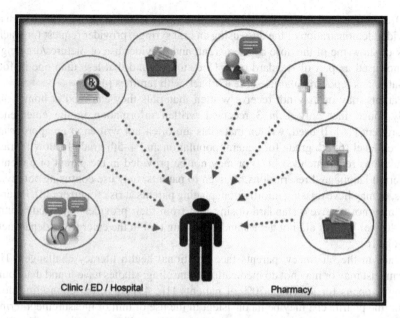

Fig. 3.3 Complexity of health literacy challenges faced by parents in understanding how to correctly administer prescription medications. *Graphic by H. Shonna Yinn*

This case highlights the potential dangers of parent misunderstanding of dosing instructions. Luckily, most cases of misunderstanding do not result in such serious consequences, but as it is difficult to know when serious errors might occur, it is best to practice universal precautions in the use of health literacy-informed communication strategies.

Understanding the challenges that families face in administering medications can be helpful for providers. The previously described health literacy challenges are cross-cutting issues for both prescription and over-the-counter (OTC) medications. For prescription medications, there are numerous additional challenges (see Fig. 3.3).

Imagine the numerous steps that a parent takes to navigate the health care system to ultimately be able to avoid a medication error. When a parent feels concerned enough to bring a sick child for evaluation in a clinical setting, whether it is to a clinic, emergency room, or other location, they are often quite stressed. Health literacy is thought to be a dynamic construct that can be influenced by environment and one's physical/mental state [44]; a stressed parent of a sick child may not be able to absorb information as clearly as they normally might [45].

When a determination that one or more medications is needed, parents often undergo verbal medication counseling from one or more health care providers (e.g. nurse, resident, attending), each of whom may provide medication instructions slightly differently. Terms like "milliliter", "teaspoon", "tablespoon", and their associated abbreviations may be used interchangeably for the same medication.

Often, effective health literacy-informed advanced counseling strategies, such as provider demonstration of the dose using an oral syringe, provider request for teach-back or show-me of the dose by the parent, and provider use of pictures/drawings, are not used as part of standard care. One study found that less than one in four pediatricians report regular use of teach-back with families [46].

Parents may or may not receive written materials they can read at home: one study found that only 1 in 3 received written information in the emergency department [16]. If used, written materials are often not written at an appropriate literacy level (6–8th grade for general population and 4–5th grade for low literacy populations recommended [47]) or may not be provided in the parent or patient's preferred language. Prescriptions, if given to parents, may use confusing abbreviations, or may have missing information, placing parents at risk for error [48]. Parents also may not receive a standard dosing tool from their provider; one study found that 80% of parents did not get a standard dosing tool in the emergency department setting [16].

Once in the pharmacy, parents face additional health literacy challenges. The pharmacist may or may not do medication counseling: studies have found that counseling happens for less than 50% of patients [16, 49]. If verbal counseling does occur, the pharmacist may be inconsistent in the use of unit of measurement terms. Or perhaps simply ask *'do you have any questions about your prescription?'* to which the patient will most likely say *'no'*.

Pharmacists may or may not give a standard dosing tool to the patient to measure the medication. Studies have found that only 20–40% of parents report received a tool in the pharmacy [19, 27]. When a tool is given in the pharmacy, the tool may often be suboptimal. Notably, few prescribed liquid medications come packaged with a dosing tool [50], and no standard guidelines exist as to which tool pharmacists should provide. Pharmacists are therefore left to make their own determination of which tool would be optimal to dispense to families. One study found that more than 30% of parents received suboptimal dosing tools that would have required them to measure multiple-instrument fills for each dose [27]; another found that just under 50% dispensed an optimal dosing tool [51]. Dosing tools also are not consistently marked with certain units of measurement, although most commonly mL is present and teaspoon is frequently included [52].

Parents face further health literacy challenges with prescription medication labels. The label on the prescription medication bottle, which is often the last place a parent or patient looks before giving a medication, is frequently poorly designed and not patient-centered [53–56]; one multi-site study found that those areas that were bolded, highlighted, and in color were not the ones most important for the parent or patient [55]. Medication instructions are typically written using times per day or hourly intervals, rather than with explicit instructions (e.g. "morning" or "night"), although there is a growing movement to improve the clarity of labels and instructions, with new guidance from groups like the US Pharmacopoeia which incorporate health literacy-informed principles [57].

Finally, written information accompanying prescription medications dispensed from the pharmacy are often written at too high of a reading level. Indeed, several studies found these materials to be at the 10–12th grade level [27, 53].

What is the result? Parents struggle to correctly administer prescribed medications. And imagine the situation where more than one medicine is prescribed. With more than one medicine being given, parents may mix up instructions. One study found that when multiple medicines were prescribed, the child had 1.6 times the odds of having a preventable adverse drug event [3].

Clearly, the health care system is not set up to make the task of dosing medication a straightforward process. Further compounding the issues described earlier is that medications that are dispensed may look different each time a prescription is filled because generic versions of the same medicines may have a different color or shape [58]. The concentration or strength of medications may be changed over time, resulting in a different volume dose to administer, presenting numeracy challenges.

Beyond dosing challenges related to units of measurement and dosing tools, parents may also have difficulty figuring out when to give their medication (e.g. does four times a day mean that a child should be woken up at night?), and for how long. They may not understand what side effects to watch out for, and when to reach out to their health care provider. Adding to these challenges is the fact that verbal counseling and written materials may not be provided in the language of parent preference [59].

Example of How Lack of Interpretation and Translation Contributed to Error

A 10-month-old girl was diagnosed with iron deficiency anemia. Her parents spoke only Spanish. No interpreter was used. The parents were counseled with broken Spanish and discharged with a prescription for iron supplements written in English. At the pharmacy, no staff spoke English and no interpreter was used—instead, the parents were counseled in English. Once home, the parents administered the medication and, within 15 min, the child vomited twice and appeared ill. Returning to the ED, the child was found to have serum iron levels 365 mcg/dL (therapeutic levels <180 mcg/dL) [60].

Health Literacy Challenges with Over-the-Counter Medications

Parents face specific health literacy challenges with over-the-counter (OTC) medications; nearly 60% of parents report difficulty understanding medication labels [61]. With OTC medications, parents often do not receive any guidance from a health care professional about which medication to give, and how much. Faced with shelves full of potential medications at the store, parents often feel overwhelmed. They must use their health literacy skills, including their document literacy skills, to deconstruct OTC medication labels. They often rely on the front panel or the "principal display panel" (PDP), and may not look at the more detailed, important information on the Drug Facts Panel [62].

When they first consider which medication to give their child, a parent must understand age restriction information. Some medications, especially cough/cold medications, are not recommended for children less than a particular age, due to potentially dangerous side effects [62]. Unfortunately, age restriction information is not mandated to be on the front panel of the medication label. Images may also serve to confuse parents regarding whether a medication should be given to their child; images of young children and teddy bears may distract parents into thinking a medication is appropriate [62]. Two studies found that the majority of parents (>50%) did not understand age restriction information and would give medications inappropriate for a child's age [62, 63].

Understanding active ingredient information is critical for recognizing when two medications have same ingredients. Such medications should not be given at the same as it increases risk of overdose. Misunderstanding of active ingredients has been linked to cases of significant morbidity, including pediatric fatalities [64]. Many parents are not able to identify the active ingredients of a medication [17, 65], and many do not understand how to use active ingredient information as part of the decision-making process [66]. Active ingredients may not be listed on the front panel of products, making it even more difficult for parents to recognize the importance of this information [66].

Example of Parent Confusion with Active Ingredient Information

A mother visited a local pharmacy to purchase several over-the-counter medicines in case her children became sick. As she was on the counter, the pharmacist asked her why she was purchasing two different brands of liquid acetaminophen. It became clear that the mother had not noticed the highlighted ingredient "acetaminophen" on the box and did not know that she was purchasing two products with same active ingredient. She could have overdosed if given together [67].

The same medications may be available in different concentrations. For example, ibuprofen comes in both infant (50 mg/1.25 mL – or 200 mg/5 mL!) and children's (100 mg/5 mL) concentrations. A parent who does not realize that the infant version is two times stronger, and knows what dose to give their child based on dosing recommendations from the "children's" version, may inadvertently give their child a two-fold overdose. Many parents perceive that an infant's medication formulation is actually weaker than a child's medication formulation [68]. Confusion between infant and children's OTC medications has led to cases of serious morbidity and mortality [6, 7]. Concerns regarding this led an FDA committee to recommend in 2009 that there should be only one version of acetaminophen. Since then, manufacturers have voluntary complied and infant acetaminophen (80 mg/0.8 mL), which is three times more concentrated than children's acetaminophen, is rarely found in the marketplace.

In the vast majority of US stores, one liquid concentration of acetaminophen predominates (160 mg/5 mL), even when it is still marketed as "infants"—with an oral syringe as measuring device included in the box, and "children's"—sold with a medicine cup as measuring device.

Confusion can also occur between adult and children's dosing: one study that compiled case reports of hepatotoxicity in children caused by multiple above the therapeutic dosing of acetaminophen found that 52% of cases in their study were caused by children receiving adult preparations of the acetaminophen [69].

Understanding the correct dose of OTC medication to give is another health literacy challenge. A dosing chart is typically included with OTC medications and parents must use their document literacy skills to navigate it. For pediatric medications such as acetaminophen and ibuprofen, dosing charts include recommendations based on both weight and age. Few parents are aware that weight rather than age should be the primary basis for dosing [12, 15], due to the wide range of weights within a given age group. Parents who know about weight-based dosing are more likely to dose correctly [15].

Finally, OTC medications are often perceived to be without side effects. Studies have found that between 27 and 88% of parents are not aware of possible side effects [17, 65, 70, 71].

Research is currently in progress to re-think OTC medication labels and to reduce the health literacy barriers for families as they seek to safely administer these medications to their families, using strategies such as color-coding and pictogram-based instructions [14, 19].

Studies of Health Literacy and Medication Errors

Conceptually, it is unsurprising that a patient's health literacy level is linked to an increased likelihood of difficulty understanding medication instructions - numerous papers in the adult literature have reached this conclusion [53, 54, 72, 73]—and a growing body of literature in pediatrics has begun to document this as well [10–13, 46, 74]. Data from the National Assessment of Adult Literacy, a nationally representative sample of US adults, found that parents with limited health literacy (below Basic or Basic health literacy) had 3.4 times the odds (95% CI: 1.6–7.4) of reporting difficulty understanding over-the-counter medication labels [61].

Parents with low health literacy may use kitchen spoons for measurement liquid medications and lack awareness of weight-based dosing [12]. Low health literacy has been linked to increased odds of making a dosing error (AOR = 1.7; 95% CI, 1.1–2.8) [11]. Parents with low health literacy are much less likely to use active ingredient information correctly [66].

It is extremely important to identify systems-based strategies aimed to overcome the health literacy barriers faced by many patients and their families in order to decrease medication errors and promote safety for pediatric patients.

Reducing Medication Errors: Counseling Strategies

Use of a health literacy-informed approach to medication counseling as part of a universal precautions approach can enhance parental understanding of medication instructions and reduce medication errors. Strategies recommended to use during medication counseling include: teach-back and show-back, dose demonstration, and use of drawings/pictures for patient education [46, 75–79].

Demonstrate, Then Confirm Understanding with Teach-Back and Show-Back

To increase the effectiveness of medication counseling, and optimize understanding of the recommended medication dose, demonstrate the correct dose with a standardized tool for parents to take home. Checking for understanding with teach-back and show-back, in concert with a dosing tool for parents to take home, may be especially effective [16]. For example, to teach a parent the appropriate dose, the provider should first show the parent the correct dose using a standard tool like an oral syringe (e.g. pulling the plunger back and pointing to the line where the correct medication dose is). Then give the 'empty' syringe to the parent and ask the parent to pull the plunger back and show-back the correct dose.

Size of Oral Syringe

For liquid medications, consider the size or capacity of the tool [27]. It is best to choose the smallest syringe to fit the dose (e.g. 5 mL syringe for a 4 mL dose), and a syringe that allows to measure the correct dose once, instead of multiple instrument-full (e.g. a 10 mL syringe for a 7.5 mL dose, rather than a 5 mL syringe) so there is no need to measure 5 mL plus 2.5 mL for the 7.5 mL dose.

When providing dosing instructions it is important to be consistent with language. A recent AAP Policy Statement endorses a move to mL-only, and elimination of teaspoon and tablespoon terms, as a strategy to decrease multifold errors and encourage the use of standard dosing tools, rather than kitchen spoons. Therefore, consider using mL only as part of verbal counseling, print instructions, and dosing instruments.

Using Drawings, Pictures and Printed Information for Patient Education

Using low literacy medication instruction sheets support verbal medication counseling. The use of both verbal and written modalities can help reinforce concepts and decrease cognitive load [80]. Parents can also refer to the written materials as they administer medications at home.

Numerous studies have documented the benefit of the use of print materials with illustrations or pictograms in improving knowledge and adherence [81, 82]; illustrated schedules have been found to assist with self-management [83, 84]. The HELPix intervention combines print materials to reinforce verbal counseling. This tool has shown to reduce parental medication errors and improve adherence to medications [19].

The HELPix includes:

1. Patient- and regimen-specific medication instruction/log sheets,
2. Provider dose demonstration with parent teach-back and show-back of the dose, and
3. Provision of standardized dosing tool (i.e. oral syringe) for liquid medications.

The instruction sheets provide a framework for medication counseling. Simple diagrams, or pictograms, reinforce information about medication dose, frequency, treatment length, preparation, and storage; a log helps parents keep track of medications. A randomized controlled trial in a New York City public hospital pediatric ED (n = 245) demonstrated the efficacy of the intervention, with decreased dosing errors (intervention vs. control: 5 vs. 48%) and non-adherence (9% vs. 38%). The instruction sheets (Fig. 3.4) were developed though Bellevue's Health Education and Literacy for Parents project, [85] a waiting room health education program. While this tool is not yet available for widespread use, generic HELPix sheets are available in the AAP book "Plain Language Pediatrics" as well as online [85, 86].

Providers who do not have access to print materials to support counseling can create their own instruction sheets by drawing pictures of dosing tools filled to the correct dose and creating regimen-specific logs for families. The log used in HELPix incorporates pictograms (e.g. sun, moon), and also has places to indicate a specific time that a dose might be given. Providers work with parents to talk about the best timing of medications convenient to the family schedules.

Summary of Medication Counseling Strategies

- Use a standard tool (e.g. oral syringe)
- Choose smallest tool to fit the dose (e.g. 5 mL syringe for 4 mL dose)
- Choose big enough tool to measure dose once (e.g. 10 mL for 7.5 mL dose)
- Show patient/caregiver the dose using the standard tool
- Ask patient/caregiver to show back the dose using the standard tool
- Use print materials with simple pictures along with verbal counseling
- Use online evidence based print materials such as those in HELPix available at http://www.med.nyu.edu/helpix/helpix-intervention/instructions-providers

Brown Bag Review and Medication Reconciliation

Medication reconciliation is another way to ensure medication safety, especially with chronic medications. This is a recommended practice across health systems [87], and involves a systematic approach to checking the medications a child is taking at each visit.

Name: _____ **Thomas** _____   **Nombre:** _____ **Thomas** _____

Information on your prescription for: Información sobre su receta para:

| **Amoxicillin**
250MG/5ML | **Amoxicillin**
250MG/5ML |

To treat an infection of the throat   Para tratar una infección de la garganta

| **7.5 mL (1½ teaspoons) by mouth**
3 times a day for 14 days | **7.5 mL (1½ cucharaditas) por la boca**
3 veces al día por 14 días |

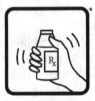
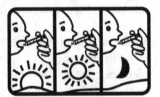
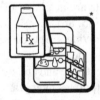

Shake well   Take **3 times a day** by mouth   Store in refrigerator
Agite bien   Tome **3 veces al día** por la boca   Guarde en la nevera

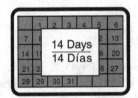
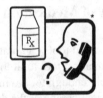

Give this medicine for 14 days,   If you have questions call
even if your child is feeling better   **(212) 562-5524** day or night
Dé esta medicina por 14 días,   Si tiene preguntas llame
aunque su niño se sienta mejor   **(212) 562-5524** día o noche

Fig. 3.4 Example of plain language, patient- and regimen-specific HELPix medication instruction sheets available online at http://www.med.nyu.edu/helpix/helpix-intervention/instructions-providers. (Accessed by H. Shonna Yin on 05/27/2016)

Keeping track of Thomas's Amoxicillin	Anotando las dosis de Thomas de Amoxicillin
7.5 mL (1½ teaspoons) by mouth 3 times a day for 14 days	**7.5 mL (1½ cucharaditas) por la boca 3 veces al día por 14 días**

❋ Date of first dose **May 12, 2008**

Parents: Please check (√) the correct box each time you give your child the medicine, 42 checks (√) total.

Fecha de la primera dosis **Mayo 12, 2008**

Padres: Por favor, marquen con (√) la casilla correcta cada vez que den la medicina a su niño, total de 42 marcas (√).

DAY / DIA	☀ (rising sun)	☀ (sun)	🌙 (moon)
Time/Hora:			
Monday / Lunes			
Tuesday / Martes			
Wednesday / Miércoles			
Thursday / Jueves			
Friday / Viernes			
Saturday / Sábado			
Sunday / Domingo			
Monday / Lunes			
Tuesday / Martes			
Wednesday / Miércoles			
Thursday / Jueves			
Friday / Viernes			
Saturday / Sábado			
Sunday / Domingo			
Monday / Lunes			

❋ Pediatrician: Please circle the starting dose and ending dose.

Fig. 3.4 continued

The AHRQ recommends reconciliation using a "Brown Bag Review." [88] The "Brown Bag Review" entails having a parent or patient bring in all the medications a child is on—including any prescription medications (e.g. liquids, pills, drops, and creams) and as-needed medications, vitamins, supplements, and herbal medications.

A designated clinic staff member should be responsible to review and discuss each medication, taking the opportunity to answer questions, verify the medicines that the patient is taking, and identify any errors or barriers to taking the medications. Review of medications may lead a physician to simplify medication regimens by reducing the number of medications or changing the schedule of medications. Providers should then provide an updated list of medications to the patient. Medication review can play an important role in ensuring patient safety and can be billed for through insurance.

References

1. Vernacchio L, Kelly J, Kaufman D, Mitchell A. Medication use among children <12 years of age in the United States: results from the Slone Survey. Pediatrics. 2009;124(2):446–54.
2. Smith M, Spiller H, Casavant M, Chounthirath T, Brophy T, Xiang H. Out-of-hospital medication errors among young children in the United States, 2002-2012. Pediatrics. 2014;134(5):867–76.
3. Zandieh S, Goldmann D, Keohane C, Yoon C, Bates D, Kaushal R. Risk factors in preventable adverse drug events in pediatric outpatients. J Pediatr. 2008;152(2):225–31.
4. Kaushal R, Goldmann D, Keohane C, et al. Adverse drug events in pediatric outpatients. Ambul Pediatr. 2007;7(5):383–9.
5. Kang A, Brooks D. US Poison control center calls for infants 6 months of age and younger. Pediatrics. 2016;137(2):1–7.
6. Tzimenatos L, Bond G, Pediatric Therapeutic Error Study G. Severe injury or death in young children from therapeutic errors: a summary of 238 cases from the American Association of Poison Control Centers. Clin Toxicol (Phila). 2009;47(4):348–54.
7. Schillie S, Shehab N, Thomas K, Budnitz D. Medication overdoses leading to emergency department visits among children. Am J Prev Med. 2009;37(3):181–7.
8. Institute for Safe Medication Practices. Eye drops or ear drops? Don't let this common mix-up happen to you! ISMP Med Saf Alert Acute Care 2016; https://www.ismp.org/newsletters/consumer/alerts/eyesEars.asp. Accessed 26 May 2016.
9. Institute for Safe Medication Practices. "And the 'eyes have it'": Eardrops, that is... ISMP Med Saf Alert Acute Care 2006; https://www.ismp.org/newsletters/acutecare/articles/20061019.asp. Accessed 26 May 2016.
10. Yin H, Mendelsohn A, Fierman A, van Schaick L, Bazan I, Dreyer B. Use of a pictographic diagram to decrease parent dosing errors with infant acetaminophen: a health literacy perspective. Acad Pediatr. 2011;11(1):50–7.
11. Yin H, Mendelsohn A, Wolf M, et al. Parents' medication administration errors: role of dosing instruments and health literacy. Arch Pediat Adol Med. 2010;164(2):181–6.
12. Yin H, Dreyer B, Foltin G, van Schaick L, Mendelsohn A. Association of low caregiver health literacy with reported use of nonstandardized dosing instruments and lack of knowledge of weight-based dosing. Ambul Pediatr. 2007;7(4):292–8.
13. Yin H, Forbis S, Dreyer B. Health literacy and pediatric health. Curr Probl Pediatr Adolesc Health Care. 2007;37(7):258–86.
14. Frush K, Luo X, Hutchinson P, Higgins J. Evaluation of a method to reduce over-the-counter medication dosing error. Arch Pediat Adol Med. 2004;158(7):620–4.
15. Li S, Lacher B, Crain E. Acetaminophen and ibuprofen dosing by parents. Pediatr Emerg Care. 2000;16(6):394–7.
16. Yin H, Dreyer B, Moreira H, et al. Liquid medication dosing errors in children: role of provider counseling strategies. Acad Pediatr. 2014;14(3):262–70.
17. Simon H, Weinkle D. Over-the-counter medications: do parents give what they intend to give? Arch Pediat Adol Med. 1997;151(7):654–6.

18. McMahon S, Rimsza M, Bay R. Parents can dose liquid medication accurately. Pediatrics. 1997;100(3):330–3.
19. Yin H, Dreyer B, van Schaick L, Foltin G, Dinglas C, Mendelsohn A. Randomized controlled trial of a pictogram-based intervention to reduce liquid medication dosing errors and improve adherence among caregivers of young children. Arch Pediat Adol Med. 2008;162(9):814–22.
20. Winnick S, Lucas D, Hartman A, Toll D. How do you improve compliance? Pediatrics. 2005;115(6):e718–24.
21. Bond G, Woodward R, Ho M. The growing impact of pediatric pharmaceutical poisoning. J Pediatr. 2012;160(2):265–70. e261
22. Yaffe S, Bierman C, Cann H, et al. Inaccuracies in administering liquid medication. Pediatrics. 1975;56(2):327–8.
23. US Department of Health Human Services. Guidance for industry: dosage delivery devices for orally ingested OTC liquid drug products. 2011; http://www.fda.gov/downloads/Drugs/GuidanceComplianceRegulatoryInformation/Guidances/UCM188992.pdf.
24. Madlon-Kay D, Mosch F. Liquid medication dosing errors. Fam Pract. 2000;49(8):741.
25. Litovitz T. Implication of dispensing cups in dosing errors and pediatric poisonings: a report from the American Association of Poison Control Centers. Ann Pharmacother. 1992;26(7–8):917–8.
26. Wansink B, van Ittersum K. Spoons systematically bias dosing of liquid medicine. Ann Inter Med. 2010;152(1):66–7.
27. Wallace L, Keenum A, DeVoe J. Evaluation of consumer medical information and oral liquid measuring devices accompanying pediatric prescriptions. Acad Pediatr. 2010;10(4):224–7.
28. Yin H, Wolf M, Dreyer B, Sanders L, Parker R. Evaluation of consistency in dosing directions and measuring devices for pediatric nonprescription liquid medications. JAMA. 2010;304(23):2595–602.
29. Sobhani P, Christopherson J, Ambrose P, Corelli R. Accuracy of oral liquid measuring devices: comparison of dosing cup and oral dosing syringe. Ann Pharmacother. 2008;42(1):46–52.
30. Yin H, Parker R, Sanders L, et al. Effect of medication label units of measure on parent choice of dosing tool: a randomized experiment. Acad Pediatr. 2016;16(8):734–41.
31. Parker R, Wolf M, Jacobson K, Wood A. Risk of confusion in dosing Tamiflu oral suspension in children. NEJM. 2009;361(19):1912–3.
32. Gaunt M. Error-Prone Units of Measure and Device Markings. 2013; http://www.pharmacy-times.com/publications/issue/2013/September2013/Error-Prone-Units-of-Measure-and-Device-Markings. Accessed 31 May 2016.
33. Yin H, Dreyer B, Ugboaja D, et al. Unit of measurement used and parent medication dosing errors. Pediatrics. 2014;134(2):e354–61.
34. Centers for Disease Control and Prevention. The PROTECT initiative: advancing children's medication safety. 2016; http://www.cdc.gov/MedicationSafety/protect/protect_Initiative.html. Accessed 27 May 2016.
35. Paul I, Committee on Drugs. Metric units and the preferred dosing of orally administered liquid medications. Pediatrics. 2015;135(4):784–87. doi:10.1542/peds.2015-0072.
36. National Council for Prescription Drug Programs. NCPDP recommendations and guidance for standardizing the dosing designations on prescription container labels of oral liquid medications. NCPDP. March 2014;White Papers.
37. Institute for Safe Medication Practices. ISMP Quarterly Action Agenda, October–December 2011. 2011; http://www.ismp.org/Newsletters/acutecare/articles/A1Q12Action.asp. Accessed 27 May 2016.
38. American Association of Poison Control Centers. AAPCC resolution - standardizing volumetric measures for oral medications intended for use by children. In: NCPDP White Papers, 2014: American Association of Poison Control Centers;2010.
39. Institute for Safe Medication Practices. Time for a change to metric. ISMP Med Saf Alert Acute Care 2006; http://www.ismp.org/Newsletters/ambulatory/archives/200604_1.asp. Accessed 31 May 2016.

40. Institute for Safe Medication Practices. ISMP calls for elimination of "Teaspoonful" and other non-metric measurements to prevent errors. 2009; http://www.ismp.org/pressroom/newsre-leases.asp.

41. Vawter S, Ralph E. The international metric system and medicine. JAMA. 1971;218(5):723–6.

42. Joint Commission. Preventing pediatric medication errors. 2008; Issue 39. https://www.joint-commission.org/sentinel_event_alert_issue_39_preventing_pediatric_medication_errors/. Accessed 27 May 2016.

43. Heubi J. Confusion with acetaminophen. 2006; https://psnet.ahrq.gov/webmm/case/115. Accessed 31 May 2016.

44. Paasche-Orlow M, Wolf M. The causal pathways linking health literacy to health outcomes. Am J Health Behav. 2007;31(Supplement 1):S19–26.

45. Yin H, Jay M, Maness L, Zabar S, Kalet A. Health literacy: an educationally sensitive patient outcome. J Gen Int Med. 2015;30(9):1363–8.

46. Turner T, Cull W, Bayldon B, et al. Pediatricians and health literacy: descriptive results from a national survey. Pediatrics. 2009;124(Supplement 3):S299–305.

47. Wallace L, Lennon E. American Academy of Family Physicians patient education materials: can patients read them? Fam Med. 2004;36(8):571–4.

48. Kaushal R, Kern L, Barron Y, Quaresimo J, Abramson E. Electronic prescribing improves medication safety in community-based office practices. J Gen Intern Med. 2010;25(6):530–6.

49. Feifer R, Greenberg L, Rosenberg-Brandl S, Franzblau-Isaac E. Pharmacist counseling at the start of therapy: patient receptivity to offers of in-person and subsequent telephonic clinical support. Popul Health Manag. 2010;13(4):189–93.

50. Johnson A, Meyers R. Evaluation of measuring devices packaged with prescription oral liquid medications. J Pediatr Pharmacol Ther. 2016;21(1):75–80.

51. Gildon B, Condren M, Phillips C, Votruba A, Swar S. Appropriateness of oral medication delivery devices available in community pharmacies. J Am Pharm Assoc (2003). 2016;56(2):137–40. e131

52. Honey B, Condren M, Phillips C, Votruba A. Evaluation of oral medication delivery devices provided by community pharmacies. Clin Pediatr (Phila). 2013;52(5):418–22.

53. Wolf M, Davis T, Tilson H, Bass P, Parker R. Misunderstanding of prescription drug warning labels among patients with low literacy. Am J Health Syst Pharm. 2006;63(11):1048–55.

54. Davis T, Wolf M, Bass P, et al. Literacy and misunderstanding prescription drug labels. Ann Inter Med. 2006;145(12):887–94.

55. Shrank W, Agnew-Blais J, Choudhry N, et al. The variability and quality of medication container labels. Arch Int Med. 2007;167(16):1760–5.

56. Shrank W, Avorn J, Rolon C, Shekelle P. Effect of content and format of prescription drug labels on readability, understanding, and medication use: a systematic review. Ann Pharmacother. 2007;41(5):783–801.

57. U.S. Pharmacopeial Convention. Prescription container labeling. 2012; United States Pharmacopoeia and National Formulary (USP 36-NF 31) http://www.usp.org/sites/default/files/usp_pdf/EN/USPNF/key-issues/c17.pdf. Accessed 26 May 2016.

58. Greene J, Kesselheim A. Why do the same drugs look different? Pills, trade dress, and public health. NEJM. 2011;365(1):83–9.

59. Bailey S, Pandit A, Curtis L, Wolf M. Availability of Spanish prescription labels: a multi-state pharmacy survey. Med Care. 2009;47(6):707–10.

60. Flores G. Language barrier. 2006; https://psnet.ahrq.gov/webmm/case/123/language-barrier. Accessed 31 May 2016.

61. Yin H, Johnson M, Mendelsohn A, Abrams M, Sanders L, Dreyer B. The health literacy of parents in the United States: a nationally representative study. Pediatrics. 2009;124(Suppl 3):S289–98.

62. Lokker N, Sanders L, Perrin E, et al. Parental misinterpretations of over-the-counter pediatric cough and cold medication labels. Pediatrics. 2009;123(6):1464–71.

63. Eiland L, Salazar M, English T. Caregivers' perspectives when evaluating nonprescription medication utilization in children. Clin Pediatr (Phila). 2008;47(6):578–87.
64. Dart R, Paul I, Bond G, et al. Pediatric fatalities associated with over the counter (nonprescription) cough and cold medications. Ann Emerg Med. 2009;53(4):411–7.
65. Birchley N, Conroy S. Parental management of over-the-counter medicines. Paediatr Nurs. 2002;14(9):24–8.
66. Yin H, Mendelsohn A, Nagin P, van Schaick L, Cerra M, Dreyer B. Use of active ingredient information for low socioeconomic status parents' decision-making regarding cough and cold medications: role of health literacy. Acad Pediatr. 2013;13(3):229–35.
67. Institute for Safe Medication Practices. All is not as it seems... When a well-known medicine does not contain what you think it contains. Horsham, PA: Institute for Safe Medication Practices; 2011.
68. Barrett T, Norton V. Parental knowledge of different acetaminophen concentrations for infants and children. Acad Emerg Med. 2000;7(6):718–21.
69. Heubi J, Barbacci M, Zimmerman H. Therapeutic misadventures with acetaminophen: hepatoxicity after multiple doses in children. J Pediatr. 1998;132(1):22–27.
70. Linder N, Sirota L, Snapir A, et al. Parental knowledge of the treatment of fever in children. Isr Med Assoc J. 1999;1(3):158–60.
71. Walsh A, Edwards H, Fraser J. Over-the-counter medication use for childhood fever: a cross-sectional study of Australian parents. J Paediatr Child Health. 2007;43(9):601–6.
72. Oates D, Paasche-Orlow M. Health literacy: communication strategies to improve patient comprehension of cardiovascular health. Circulation. 2009;119(7):1049–51.
73. Rothman R, Yin H, Mulvaney S, Co J, Homer C, Lannon C. Health literacy and quality: focus on chronic illness care and patient safety. Pediatrics. 2009;124:S315–26.
74. Tanner S, Wells M, Scarbecz M, McCann Sr B. Parents' understanding of and accuracy in using measuring devices to administer liquid oral pain medication. J Am Dent Assoc. 2014;145(2):141–9.
75. Weiss L, Gany F, Rosenfeld P, et al. Access to multilingual medication instructions at New York City pharmacies. J Urban Health. 2007;84(6):742–54.
76. Dowse R, Ehlers M. Medicine labels incorporating pictograms: do they influence understanding and adherence? Patient Educ Couns. 2005;58(1):63–70.
77. Schwartzberg J, Cowett A, VanGeest J, Wolf M. Communication techniques for patients with low health literacy: a survey of physicians, nurses, and pharmacists. Am J Health Behav. 2007;31(Supplement 1):S96–S104.
78. Joint Commission. "What did the doctor say?": improving health literacy to protect patient safety. In: Report Health Care at the Crossroads reports, 2017.
79. Paasche-Orlow M, Schillinger D, Greene S, Wagner E. How health care systems can begin to address the challenge of limited literacy. J Gen Int Med. 2006;21(8):884–7.
80. Pusic M, Ching K, Yin H, Kessler D. Seven practical principles for improving patient education: evidence-based ideas from cognition science. Paediatr Child Health. 2014;19(3):119.
81. Katz M, Kripalani S, Weiss B. Use of pictorial aids in medication instructions: a review of the literature. Am J Health Syst Pharm. 2006;63(23):2391–7.
82. Houts P, Doak C, Doak L, Loscalzo M. The role of pictures in improving health communication: a review of research on attention, comprehension, recall, and adherence. Patient Educ Couns. 2006;61(2):173–90.
83. Schillinger D, Machtinger E, Wang F, Palacios J, Rodriguez M, Bindman A. Language, literacy, and communication regarding medication in an anticoagulation clinic: a comparison of verbal vs. visual assessment. J Health Commun. 2006;11(7):651–64.
84. Morrow D, Hier C, Menard W, Leirer V. Icons improve older and younger adults' comprehension of medication information. J Gerontol B Psychol Sci Soc Sci. 1998;53(4):P240–54.
85. HELPIX. Instruction for providers. http://www.med.nyu.edu/helpix/helpix-intervention/instructions-providers. Accessed 27 May 2016.

86. Abrams M, Dreyer B. Plain language pediatrics. AAP Books Elk Grove Village, IL. 2008.
87. Joint Commission. Issue 35: using medication reconciliation to prevent errors. 2006; https://www.jointcommission.org/assets/1/18/SEA_35.pdf
88. Agency for Healthcare Research and Quality. Conduct Brown Bag Medicine Reviews: Tool #8. February 2015; http://www.ahrq.gov/professionals/quality-patient-safety/quality-resources/tools/literacy-toolkit/healthlittoolkit2-tool8.html

Chapter 4
Health Literacy Universal Precautions: Strategies for Communication with All Patients

Rosina Avila Connelly and Aditi Gupta

Universal Precautions

"I speak to everyone in the same way, whether he is the garbage man or the president of the university."

—Albert Einstein

We have already discussed the state of low health literacy, affecting up to 90 million Americans. Almost 90% of adults may be affected by low health literacy, with only 12% of adults demonstrating proficient literacy skills (NAAL 2006). Clinicians cannot tell by looking which patient is the one in ten who will have proficient literacy skills and, hence, should use the universal precaution approach to low health literacy by implementing strategies for clear communication with *all* patients.

This chapter will discuss simple but practical health literacy strategies for communication which should be used with all patients. These strategies include tips for effective verbal communication and for effective use of written communication.

Strategies for Verbal Communication

"The two words 'information' and 'communication' are often used interchangeably, but they signify quite different things. Information is giving out; communication is getting through."

—Sydney J. Harris

R.A. Connelly (✉)
Division of General Pediatrics, Department of Pediatrics & Adolescent Medicine, University of South Alabama, Mobile, AL, USA
e-mail: rosinaconnelly@health.southalabama.edu

A. Gupta, DO
Department of Pediatrics, Baylor College of Medicine, 6621 Fannin Street, Clinical Care Center, Suite 1540.00, Houston, TX 77030-2399, USA

© The Editor(s) and The Author(s) 2017   39
R.A. Connelly, T. Turner (eds.), *Health Literacy and Child Health Outcomes*, SpringerBriefs in Public Health, DOI 10.1007/978-3-319-50799-6_4

Avoid Using Medical Jargon

One important strategy for improving verbal communication with patients is to eliminate medical jargon. Jargon is defined as "the technical terminology or characteristic idiom of a special activity or group." [1] Medical jargon, then, is the technical language of medicine. Imagine you are in another country where the predominant language is something other than English. How do would you feel listening to other people talk in a language you do not understand? This is how someone with low health literacy feels when talking with a healthcare provider who uses medical jargon. Many of these patients feel frustrated and confused because they cannot understand what the healthcare provider is saying. They may also feel embarrassed to ask questions. By eliminating medical jargon from their conversations, healthcare providers can better communicate with patients and their families.

The Institute of Medicine (IOM) defines patient-centered care as: "providing care that is respectful of and responsive to individual patient preferences, needs, and values, and ensuring that patient values guide all clinical decisions." [2] Practicing patient-centered care allows the physician to tailor the care plan around characteristics specific to the patient rather than simply the disease process. It involves using a style of communication that gives the patient or family a larger role in the patient-doctor interaction and in the decision-making process [2].

How do we avoid using medical jargon? Numerous strategies and resources are available to aid in this process, but communication begins by using simple terms [3] and practicing patient-centered care [2] that allows the patient to have a stake in the decision-making process.

Use Plain Language

Healthcare providers can keep things simple by using everyday words or "plain language." The Plain Language Information and Action Network, a group of federal employees who advocate for clarity of language in the government, describes plain language as communication *your audience* can understand the first time it is read or heard. Language that is plain to one audience may not be plain to others. Plain language is defined by results—it is easy to read, understand, and use [3].

Substituting simple words for jargon is the first step towards better communication, but one must still make sure that a patient understands the simpler words. We will discuss checking for understanding later in this chapter. One good resource to help with using simpler language is the *Plain Language Thesaurus* that has been compiled by the Centers for Disease Control and Prevention's National Center for Health Marketing [4]. It offers plain-language equivalents to medical terms, phrases, and references commonly used by healthcare providers [4].

Patients have expressed their need for health care providers to use simpler words and to check for understanding.

One study in Poland analyzed interviews at a tertiary care medical center to determine how pediatric patients and their parents perceive health care during hospital stays, what their expectations of doctors' behaviors are, and which components of care they consider to be the most important. Two themes emerged from the authors' analysis. One involved doctors' verbal and non-verbal behaviors, which included informing and explaining, discussing topics other than the illness, tone of voice, and other behaviors. The other theme involved perceived strategies used by doctors. Use of medical jargon was prevalent in both themes, as observed by the following examples.

Some patients thought that physicians use medical jargon because they have limited time to interact with the patient.

> "It's hard to inform someone who knows nothing about medicine, isn't it? This is the problem: using words and terms which mean nothing to us. And the Latin expressions sound like magic charms. Basically, we don't know what they are talking about. So it's important to transform the information to a level understandable for an average mother or father. … It requires patience and time, first of all, time" (mother of a 5-year-old boy, age 45, higher education).

Other patients expressed their opinion that physicians used medical jargon purposefully to limit the conversation with the patient or to avoid answering the patient's questions.

> "If the doctor tries to explain something, he or she uses a lot of specialist terms; often the parents have to guess what they mean. They often avoid the answer. Maybe they don't want to make the patient worry or maybe for another reason. They avoid it by using very specialist words. And they succeed. … If I don't understand, I ask. I often ask but they [doctors] ignore certain subjects. So I've come to understand that if doctors use such specialized language, they are trying to avoid telling me something." (Father of a 4-month-old child, age 25, higher education) [5].

By avoiding the use of jargon, healthcare providers can create an environment that empowers and encourages patients to ask questions and that better ensures understanding of information for all patients.

> "I know that you believe you understand what you think I said, but I am not sure you realize that what you heard is not what I meant."
>
> —Robert McCloskey

Check for Understanding: Teach-Back and Show-Me Techniques

Another important strategy for improving verbal communication with patients is to check for understanding. Studies have shown that 40–80% of the medical information patients receive is forgotten immediately [6] and nearly half of the information retained is incorrect [7]. In a busy practice, physicians often assess understanding by asking *"Do you understand?"* or *"Do you have any questions?"* Imagine you are a patient who has no idea what your doctor just told you. Your doctor has just spent 10 min explaining a concept to you and is about to leave and then asks you one of the above questions. Would you feel comfortable saying "yes, I have questions" or "no, I do not understand"?

Teach-Back Technique

One of the easiest ways to close the gap in communication between clinician and patient is to employ the "teach-back" method or "closing the loop." [8] The teach-back process involves asking a patient to explain back to you in his or her own words the information that you just provided. Teach-back is not a test of the patient's knowledge; rather it is a test of how well you explained the information to the patient [9]. Some approaches that can be used when using teach-back include the following:

1. We talked a lot about diet and exercise changes today and I want to make sure I communicated it well. What diet changes are you going to focus on for the next 2 months? What exercise changes are you going to focus on?
2. How are you going to give this medication to your child at home? Ok, how often will you give it? Ok, for how long will you give it?
3. How would you explain to your husband the information we discussed today?

Using teach-back involves several steps. The first step is to solicit teach-back using a prompt such as one of the above. It is important when doing so to ask the parents or patient to explain the information using his or her own words. When families repeat information back verbatim, it is difficult to assess whether they understood it or simply stored the words in their short-term memory. In the second step, the healthcare provider listens to the patient's or parent's answer to assess whether she understood the information. If the patient is unable to explain the information, the next step is to explain the information again, this time using different words.

Once again, check for understanding. If the patient is still unable to explain it, consider using a different strategy to explain the information but continue using teach-back to assess whether they understand it [9].

In order to become comfortable with using teach-back, it is important to practice it with every patient, whether or not you perceive that the patient is struggling to understand [9].

Teach-back can be used with any type of medical information. It is most commonly used when counseling families about medication use or lifestyle changes. For example, teach-back is often used to ask patients or parents to explain back to the physician how often or for how long they will need to take a particular medication. It can also be used with lifestyle changes, including diet and exercise goals, as well as any other information that the healthcare provider needs to impart, such as signs or symptoms that may occur.

Numerous studies have demonstrated the effectiveness of teach-back [10–11]. One study specifically looked at its use in the hospital discharge process. In this study, nurses learned the teach-back process, implemented it with patients, and then answered survey questions regarding ease of use and effectiveness of the process [10]. When asked to comment on teach-back, staff remarked that it was "useful, valuable, simple, a great idea, and something everyone should use." Nurses were also asked if by using teach-back, they were able to clarify information and correct some misunderstandings that they would not have been able to do otherwise. More than half responded, "yes." They identified misunderstandings about medication administration and measurement, formula dilution, and follow-up appointment scheduling as areas in which they were able to correct misunderstandings [10].

Another study done in Jamaica assessed maternal health literacy of pregnant women and evaluated their ability to communicate the benefits, risks, and safety of specific vaccines after using the teach-back method. The authors found that health literacy scores were moderately, positively correlated with identification of vaccine risks and benefits. Thus, teach-back was more effective with women who had higher health literacy [11].

Although teach-back has been shown to be an effective way of communicating with families, in a qualitative study interviewing both adult patients and parents of pediatric patients in an emergency room setting, interviewees revealed concerns about the use of teach-back. Many interviewees, particularly those with limited health literacy, responded that teach-back techniques could easily be seen as condescending, judgmental, and reinforcing existing power differentials between patients and providers. Several interviewees thought that this would occur only if teach-back was introduced inappropriately, and they provided suggestions on wording and ideas to introduce teach-back that would be less likely to be seen as offensive. They included recognizing the potential for teach-back to be seen as insulting, and addressing that concern in the introduction, explaining that often people forget information after leaving the ED, and focusing on the potential for the provider to have explained something incorrectly as being the justification for teach-back [12].

Show-Me Technique

The show-me technique is similar to teach-back but it involves the parent showing the health care provider how to do something rather than just explaining it [9]. This strategy can be especially useful with administration of medication [9]. For example, a parent may need to give a patient 4 mL of an antibiotic twice a day. You can use teach-back to make sure the mother understands the dose of the medication and how often she should give it, but it does not help with the actual act of measuring the medication into the syringe. By using the show-me technique, you can have the mother use a syringe and measure 4 mL of liquid. Incorporating both the show-me and teach-back techniques allows for a greater overall understanding of the concept.

The show-me technique is commonly used with asthma education, specifically for use of the inhaler and spacer. Families often do not understand how to use an inhaler correctly, which can compromise the effectiveness of the medication. By having a patient or parent demonstrate the technique rather than merely explain how to do it, a healthcare provider can better assess the patient's understanding [9].

In summary, teach-back and show-me techniques are strategies that healthcare providers can use to assess a patient or parent's understanding of medical information. In order for either technique to be effective, it needs to be introduced in a way that avoids judgment and makes people feel comfortable without taking offense to the questioning. It should also be used as many times as needed with a particular concept to ensure the patient or parent has demonstrated understanding.

Encourage Patients to Ask Questions

A third important strategy for improving spoken communication with patients is to encourage patients to ask questions. As with assessing understanding, it is often done in a close-ended manner by asking, *"Do you have any questions?"* Because of numerous factors, including the way questions are solicited and the nature of the doctor-patient relationship, encouraging the patient to ask questions often is unsuccessful, not because patients do not have any questions but more likely because they are uncomfortable asking them. In some cultures, patients' regard for the health care providers can curb their desire to ask questions because they perceive doing so as questioning the expertise of a person whom they hold in high regard [13].

Creating an environment that encourages patients to ask questions is essential to helping patients understand and take ownership in their health [13].

This is where "Ask Me 3" comes in handy. "Ask Me 3" was developed by the National Patient Safety Foundation. It is an educational initiative that encourages patients and families to ask three specific questions of their healthcare provider to better understand their health [14].

The three "Ask Me 3" questions are: [14]

1. What is my main problem?
2. What do I need to do?
3. Why is it important for me to do this?

Patients can use the Ask Me 3 questions to become more involved in the provider-patient conversation and to be more focused on the information they need to take care of their health. Providers can also use the questions asked in the Ask Me 3 program to help structure their patient visits [14].

Creating an environment that encourages questions can also have lasting effects on a clinic or practice by decreasing the number of phone calls the clinic receives from patients to clarify information. It can also increase both patient satisfaction and patient safety, all of which lead to better care for patients [13].

Implementing Ask Me 3 should be a group effort that includes everyone working in the healthcare field. From the receptionist at the front desk to the physician seeing the patient, all have a part in implementing Ask Me 3. At the front desk, brochures and posters explaining Ask Me 3 can be useful in giving the patient the idea of asking questions. When vitals are being taken and a chief complaint elicited, Ask Me 3 can be used by the clinical staff to encourage the patient to ask questions of the physician. The physician seeing the patient can use Ask Me 3 to help structure the visit. Lastly, at checkout, the desk clerk could ask the patient whether their questions were answered.

Along with soliciting questions in a clinic setting, Ask Me 3 should be used to solicit questions from other health care providers, including nurses, therapists, and pharmacists. Primary-care physicians have the responsibility to encourage and empower patients to ask questions about all aspects of their health, whether in the primary care physician's office or another healthcare setting.

Studies evaluating the effectiveness of Ask Me 3 in pediatrics are scarce. One study done in family practice clinics with adult patients asked the following questions:

1. Does the Ask Me 3 intervention affect patients' question-asking behavior?
2. Does the Ask Me 3 intervention affect adherence to selected physicians' treatment recommendations?
3. Is there a relationship between patient question-asking, in general, and these same adherence outcomes?

They found that the Ask Me 3 intervention did not increase the frequency of patients' question-asking, either for the Ask Me 3 questions specifically or for questions generally. The Ask Me 3 intervention also did not improve patients' adherence to treatment recommendations. The authors suggested that these findings resulted from a high level of baseline questioning they found in their patients; hence, after implementing Ask Me 3, a ceiling effect occurred and a significant number of new questions were not asked [15]. Another study looked specifically at the implementation of Ask Me 3 in a pediatric outpatient clinic. The researchers found that 6 months after a simple implementation of Ask Me 3 in their practice, at least 20% of patients were still using it [16].

In summary, Ask Me 3 seeks to encourage patients to ask questions in order to better understand their health. By implementing Ask Me 3 in a variety of healthcare settings, healthcare providers can empower patients and parents to ask questions in order to better understand and take control over their health [13].

Limit the Amount of Information and Repeat: Chunk and Check

A fourth important strategy for improving verbal communication with patients is to limit the amount of information being disseminated at one time. As previously mentioned, studies have shown that 40–80% of the medical information patients receive is forgotten immediately [6] and nearly half of the information retained is incorrect [7]. Reinforcement of information is essential for retention. When patients come for visits with their healthcare providers, they are often bombarded with a large amount of information pertaining to different aspects of their health. Patients can easily become overwhelmed when so much information given to them at one time.

One strategy used to overcome these issues is called "Chunk and Check", often used along with teach-back to help patients understand information. It involves three simple steps:

The first step: Break down the information that needs to be discussed into manageable chunks [17]. The U.S. Department of Health and Human Services recommends limiting conversations to four main messages [18].

The second step: Give one chunk of information using plain language [17].

The third step: Stop and assess for understanding before moving on to the next chunk of information. This is the "check" step [17] in which, instead of soliciting questions and assessing understanding at the *end* of the visit, the physician does so numerous times *during* the visit, after delivering each 'chunk' of information.

It is important to consider the order in which to deliver the "chunk" of information. Consider giving the most important information first. "Chunk and check" helps patients understand information better because it encourages questions. When patients wait until the end of the visit to ask questions, either because they do not want to interrupt the physician or because they do not have a chance to ask, they forget their questions and/or the physician does not have as much time to sit and discuss the answers. By encouraging questions after each chunk of information is imparted, we can make sure patients' questions are answered in a way that maximizes their understanding [17].

> *"Many attempts to communicate are nullified by saying too much."*
>
> —Robert Greenleaf

Strategies for Written Information: Using Pictures and Models and Written Information Effectively

> *"A picture is worth a thousand words"*
>
> —American Idiom

Effectiveness of written health communication has been mentioned in previous chapters and will be discussed in Chap. 5, in the context of using plain language and patient-centered approach to communication for creating a patient-friendly and shame-free environment. More importantly, Chap. 5 will discuss the importance of using plain language in written information and other recommendations for effective written health communication with all patients.

Using Pictures and Models: Patient Education

Clinicians are educators to parents and patients. Drawing knowledge from human cognitive theories and evidence-based ideas from cognition science, Pusic et al. provided recommendations for improved patient education [19]. Cognitive load, dual code and multimedia theories provide the basis for their recommendations to improve patient education as follows:

1. Bypass working memory—use printed information instead of relying on verbal recall
2. Patient to control flow of information—check for understanding
3. Limit cognitive load—use simple drawings, focus on the need to know
4. Use multiple senses for learning—present verbal information and pictures or graphics and do so at the same time, to combine visual and aural information for best uptake
5. Leave out extraneous or unnecessary information—less is more

Patients and parents have a very limited amount of time during the clinical encounter to convey information, undergo examination and appropriate testing or procedures needed for diagnosis. The clinician delivers a diagnosis and gives instructions sometimes for multiple tasks, each with several steps, for the patient to carry on after the visit. When patients do not have questions, clinicians assume that communication has taken place and feel reassured at the end of the visit by handing out a computer-generated patient plan. Only to be baffled at the fact that, for whatever reason, the patient did not follow instructions, or worse—a medication error resulted in worsening of the initial condition.

Here is an anecdote to illustrate how bad communication happens to people with the best intentions to practice effective health communication:

A 9-month old infant, who has had a congenital heart defect repair and has taken medications on a daily basis, is diagnosed with ear infection. Clinician gave information to include medication dose and importance of using the syringe to measure the correct amount of the antibiotic. The mother stated there were no questions at the end of the visit, and declined a printed patient plan due to having to leave the in a hurry. Patient returned with symptoms of vomiting after every dose of antibiotic 48 h after his initial visit. When clinician—who relied in the mother's previous experience with giving heart medications and made assumption that patient's mother would recall all instructions—asked for how much antibiotic had been given to the child, the answer was '5 mL, just as you told me'.

But the chart clearly indicated dose was 2 mL and that is how it was written in the script. The mother had the bottle with her—great brown bag review and medication reconciliation strategy—and pointed out where she found instructions for 5 mL on the label. Only that she had looked at the area with the name and concentration 'Cefprozil 250 mg/5 mL' and not the area with the actual medication instructions 'TAKE 2 MILLILITERS BY MOUTH EVERY 12 HOURS FOR 10 DAYS' [see Fig. 4.1].

What could have the clinician done differently to ensure patient education was not tainted by health literacy and cognitive overload barriers?

1. Use universal precautions: even though the patient's mother had given liquid heart medications to her baby earlier in life, the clinician should recognize that every encounter brings new information and not presume the mother would understand right away.

Fig. 4.1 This patient's mother should have left the office with a standard medication syringe after verbal counseling and demonstrations. *Photo: Rosina Avila Connelly*

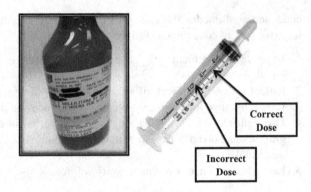

2. Use a model: the clinician should take an oral medication syringe and demonstrate that for this medication, an antibiotic, she should measure 2 mL and mark the 2 mL-line in the syringe.
3. Check for understanding: the clinician should give the syringe to the mother and ask her to show on the syringe how much medication her child needs.
4. Give written information with the key messages: your child has an ear infection; give your child 2 mL of antibiotic 'cefprozil' in the morning and in the evening; give for 10 days.

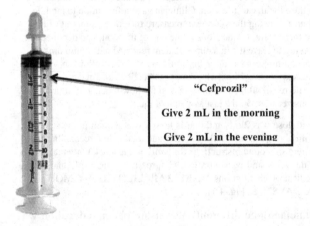

Using Written Materials and Pictures for Effective Patient Education

Written information for effective patient education involves more than plain language to effectively result in learning that leads to behavior change. [19] A study by Davis et al. showed that using plain language and simply written patient education handouts significantly improved understanding of health information—but only for participants with good reading skills—as participants who read poorly did not benefit much from easy-to-read materials [20]. Adding pictures to easy-to-read written information improved health communication in another study, as participants were 1.5 times more likely to correctly answer questions related to the health information given at the end of the visit [20].

Interestingly, the types of pictures used to accompany written information greatly impact the learning process and the ability to understand written health information. Delp and Jones found that simple cartoon drawings were more effective than matchstick figures and photographs [21]. A combination of text and simple drawings or pictures mean less cognitive load and has been very helpful for individuals with low health literacy skills [19, 21]. Using pictures when giving written information to patients increases recall of verbal instructions [22]. Furthermore, pictures should be meaningful to the audience, and culturally relevant, as emotional response has been found to affect behavior change [23].

Recommendations for Using Pictures in Health Education

Houts et al. provided a summary of recommendations for the use of pictures and written information when communicating with patients [23].

- Patient information should include pictures to facilitate health communication
- Use the simplest drawings or photographs possible
- Point at pictures while giving verbal information
- Written text should be clear, using plain language
- Information written should be relevant, culturally sensitive
- Leaving white space between photos and texts increases clarity
- Health educators should be involved in the design and evaluation of health written material

In summary, written information that incorporate simple drawings or graphics, and is given along with verbal instructions provide visual and auditory stimuli that facilitates learning. Giving simple written instructions with drawings also decreases the barriers of cognitive overload and deficient working memory during patient education in a brief clinical encounter. Let the patients decide the flow of, and amount of information, allowing them to process the verbal and visual stimuli when acquiring new knowledge. The extra time taken during one encounter will result in time savings in the future by ensuring health communication and decreasing chances for medication errors and unnecessary use of health resources.

References

1. "Jargon." Merriam-Webster.com. Merriam-Webster, n.d. Web. 24 Apr 2016.
2. Institute of Medicine. Crossing the quality chasm: a new health system for the 21st Century Committee on Quality of Health Care in America. Washington, DC: National Academy Press; 2001.
3. Plain language: what is plain language? Plainlanguage.gov. N.p. 2016 Web 25 Apr 2016.
4. National Center for Health Marketing and the Center for Disease Control. Plain language thesaurus for health communication. Atlanta, GA: CDC; 2009.
5. Konstantynowicz J, Marcinowicz L, Abramowicz P, et al. What do children with chronic diseases and their parents think about pediatricians? A qualitative interview study. Matern Child Health J. 2016;20(8):1745–52. [Epub ahead of print]
6. Kessels RP. Patients' memory for medical information. J R Soc Med. 2003;96(5):219–22.
7. Anderson JL, Dodman S, Kopelman M, et al. Patient information recall in a rheumatology clinic. Rheumatology. 1979;18(1):18–22.
8. Schillinger D, Piette J, Grumbach K, et al. Closing the loop: physician communication with diabetic patients who have low health literacy. Arch Intern Med. 2003;163(1):83–90.
9. Brega AG, Barnard J, Mabachi NH, et al. (2015) Tool 5: the teach-back method. In: Health literacy universal precautions toolkit. 2nd ed. http://www.ahrq.gov/sites/default/files/wysiwyg/professionals/quality-patient-safety/quality-resources/tools/literacy-toolkit/healthlittoolkit2_tool5.pdf. Accessed 23 Apr 2016
10. Kornburger C, Gibson C, Sadowski S, et al. Using "Teach-Back" to promote a safe transition from hospital to home: an evidence-based approach to improving the discharge process. J Pediatr Nurs. 2013;28:282–91.
11. Wilson FL, Mayeta-Peart A, Parada-Webster L, et al. Using the teach-back method to increase maternal immunization literacy among low-income pregnant women in Jamaica: a pilot study. J Pediatr Nurs. 2012;27:451–9.
12. Samuels-Kalow M, Hardy E, Rhodes K, et al. "Like a dialogue": Teach-back in the emergency department. Patient Educ Couns. 2015;99(4):549–54.
13. Brega AG, Barnard J, Mabachi NH, et al. (2015) Tool 14: encouraging questions. In: Health literacy universal precautions toolkit. 2nd ed. http://www.ahrq.gov/sites/default/files/wysiwyg/professionals/quality-patient-safety/quality-resources/tools/literacy-toolkit/healthlittoolkit2_tool14.pdf Accessed 19 Apr 2016
14. National Patient Safety Foundation. Ask Me 3. 2016. http://www.npsf.org/?page=askme3. Accessed 19 Apr 2016.
15. Galliher JM, Post DM, Weiss BD, et al. Patients' question-asking behavior during care visits: a report from the AAFP National Research Network. Ann Fam Med. 2010;8(2):152–9.
16. Mika VS, Wood PR, Weiss BD, et al. Ask Me 3: improving communication in a Hispanic pediatric outpatient practice. Am J Health Behav. 2007;Suppl 1:S115–21.
17. The Knowledge Center. The health literacy place: chunk and check. 2016. http://wwwhealthliteracyplaceorguk/tools-and-techniques/techniques/chunk-and-check/. Accessed 17 Apr 2016.
18. US Department of Health and Human Services Quick Guide to Health Literacy. http://health.gov/communication/literacy/quickguide/Quickguide.pdf Accessed 25 Apr 2016.
19. Pusic MV, Ching K, Yin HS, Kessler D. Seven practical principles for improving patient education: evidence-based ideas from cognition science. Paediatr Child Health. 2014;19(3):119–22.
20. Davis TC, Bocchini JA, Fredrickson D, Arnold C, Mayeaux EJ, Murphy PW, Jackson RH, Hanna N, Paterson M. Parent comprehension of polio vaccine information pamphlets. Pediatrics. 1996;97(6):804–10.
21. Austin PE, Matlack R, Dunn KA, Kosler C, Brown CK. Discharge instruction: do illustrations help our patients understand them? Ann Emerg Med. 1995;25:317–20.
22. Moll JM. Doctor-patient communication in rheumatology: studies of visual and verbal perception using educational booklets and other graphic material. Ann Rheum Dis. 1986;45(3):198–209.
23. Houts PS, et al. The role of pictures in improving health communication: a review of research on attention, comprehension, recall, and adherence. Patient Educ Couns. 2005;61(2):173–19.

Chapter 5
Health Literacy and Effective Health Communication in Pediatric Practices and Health Systems: Creating Shame-Free Environments and Patient-Friendly Institutions

Aditi Gupta and Michael E. Speer

Will Patients Feel Welcome and Encouraged to Ask Questions?

Shame has been defined as a "painful emotion caused by consciousness of guilt, shortcoming, or impropriety" [1]. Several researchers have characterized patients with low literacy as being unwilling to disclose their problems to healthcare providers because of their shame [2, 3].

Contributing to this feeling of inadequacy is the reading level of most patient materials. Wilson examined 35 unique patient educational materials produced by professional sources (government agencies, drug companies, and state/national organizations) or by providers [4]. Professionally developed materials had significantly higher reading levels and were more difficult to read, but all materials were written at a reading level higher than most adults can comprehend [4]. D'Alessandro DM and co-workers reported similar results. They evaluated a hundred different web sites designed for laypersons for general readability of pediatric patient education materials designed for adults. They found that the average reading level on these websites was above the 10.6 grade level [5]. Most adult high school graduates read at the seventh to eighth grade level [6–8]. Most consent forms are written at the tenth grade level or higher [8].

A. Gupta, DO (✉)
Department of Pediatrics, Baylor College of Medicine, 6621 Fannin Street,
Clinical Care Center, Suite 1540.00, Houston, TX 77030-2399, USA
e-mail: axgupta1@texaschildrens.org

M.E. Speer, M.D.
Section of Neonatology, Department of Pediatrics, Baylor College of Medicine,
Texas Children's Hospital, 6621 Fannin St., Suite W6104 Mail Stop: MC WT6-10,
Houston, TX 77030, USA
e-mail: mspeer@bcm.edu

© The Editor(s) and The Author(s) 2017   51
R.A. Connelly, T. Turner (eds.), *Health Literacy and Child Health Outcomes*,
SpringerBriefs in Public Health, DOI 10.1007/978-3-319-50799-6_5

Creating a Shame-Free Environment Within a Patient-Friendly Institution

First and foremost, the healthcare provider must evaluate the environment that patients encounter when they present to the office, clinic, or hospital. That concern includes all of the paperwork that the parent must read such as handouts, consent and intake forms, and insurance forms. An administrative staff that can help the patients in completing forms helps immensely. Patient materials should be written at the sixth-grade level or lower [8]. Only patient-specific information that is necessary to the visit should be collected. Some questions that are helpful in evaluating the environment are: What is the atmosphere like? Is the staff exhibiting an aura of helpfulness? Are they using everyday language or *medicaleze*? Are they speaking the patient's preferred language? Do they offer to mail, fax, or e-mail a map to new patients who make enquiries rather than sending a set of complicated instructions?

The Patient-Centered Approach to Communication

The use of plain language (e.g., "high blood pressure," not "hypertension"; "heart doctor," not "cardiologist"), delivered slowly, is an imperative for comprehension to occur [9–14]. This is a conversation; a two-way exchange. Remember when using a translator to instruct him or her that your statements are to be translated into "everyday" words for the patient/parents. Given many patients' limited health literacy (e.g., 60% of Medicaid patients have literacy skills at or below the NAAL Basic category) [15], the use of medical terms causes inadequate and even confusing communication [14]. Further, patients commonly state that physicians do not explain their illness or treatment options to them in language they can comprehend [14]. From a governmental or societal perspective, this poor communication is unacceptable.

The Plain Writing Act of 2010 requires federal agencies to write "clear Government communication that the public can understand and use" [16]. Other techniques for fostering a patient-friendly environment for parents include sitting instead of standing, listening instead of talking, and asking parents if they have concerns [8].

Do not ask parents if they "understand," as they invariably answer "yes," whether they do or not [12]. Williams et al., proposed six steps to improve communication with patients:

• Spend a small amount of extra time with each patient (parent)
• Use plain, everyday language
• Use teach-back or show-me examples
• Make the environment such that the parents are comfortable asking questions

- Limit the amount of information given at any one time and repeat the same information at least once
- Show or draw pictures; pictures are indeed worth a 1000 words [17]

Some physicians are concerned that this approach will unduly lengthen the time of an office visit; this is not the case. Langewitz et al., demonstrated quite clearly that the mean spontaneous talking time by a patient was 1 min and 32 s, with a median value of 59 s [18]. Blau reported similar findings several years earlier [19].

Physicians are notorious for interrupting patients. Marvel and colleagues reported that physicians redirected the patient's opening statement after a mean of 23.1 s. Patients allowed to complete their statement regarding their reason for the physician visit used only 6 s more on average than those who were redirected. Late-arising patient concerns were more common when physicians did not solicit patients' concerns during the interview (34.9% vs 14.9%) [20]. Thus, interrupting patients/parents may actually prolong the encounter as opposed to efficiently addressing the issues.

Plain Language in Patient Information Materials: From Registration Forms, Consent Forms, and General Information, to Information Giving and Patient Education Resources

"The more elaborate our means of communication, the less we communicate."

—Joseph Priestley

Parents encounter many different forms of written communication throughout the process of taking their child to be seen by a physician. Imagine that it's Sunday, you are the parent of a 5-year-old child who has had cough and fever up to 102 for 3 days. Let's go through the steps involved in getting your child seen by a doctor.

1. You need to understand how sick your child is. Do you need to take the child to an urgent care center or to the emergency room? Or can you wait until next business day to call the doctor's office?
2. You decide to go to an urgent care center and have transportation to get there. Now you are at the front desk and are given a packet of forms to fill out. One form asks all sorts of demographic information. The other asks about your child's health history. Another asks about any medications you have given the child. The last one is a consent form for treatment.
3. You fill out the forms and wait to be seen. After some time, you are put in a room and the physician examines your child. The physician tells you that your child has pneumonia and that she needs to take antibiotics for 10 days. She tells you she will send the script for the medication to your pharmacy and tells you to follow-up with your regular pediatrician in 1–2 days.

4. You wait for your discharge paperwork and are sent home with a copy of the prescription, as well as some information about pneumonia.
5. On your way home, you stop by the pharmacy to pick up the medication for your daughter.

During these steps there were several times when written communication was used: the registration packet with all its multiple components, the discharge paperwork with information about the disease, and the prescription. Written information about the illness given probably by the nurse during the process of discharge—when oral communication is also taking place. As mention earlier, even a highly educated person will have difficulties with health literacy during a stressful situation such as the one described above. When a person with low health literacy encounters written materials, many barriers may prevent them from understanding the material. Some parents with low health literacy may not be familiar with key medical terms in the material, which can lead to misunderstanding. Other parents may not understand text written at a higher reading level. Still others may not be able to piece out the important points in the documents because they are buried in a dense amount of text [21].

So, how do we tailor that written information to those with lower health literacy? One way is by using plain language. Plain language is language that is easy to read, understand and use [22].

The Plain Language Information and Action Network offers other techniques to develop effective written materials. Some of these techniques include logical organization with the reader in mind, using 'you' and other pronouns, writing short sentences using the active voice, using common every day words, and using easy-to-read design features. Some of these design features include larger font (size 11 or 12), a certain amount of write space on the page, bulleted lists, and headings and subheadings to separate blocks of text [22].

In 2009, the American Academy of Pediatrics developed a set of 25 plain language handouts in both English and Spanish [21]. These handouts cover a range of acute, chronic, and preventive topics for different ages, and were developed taking in consideration elements of plain language when developing these forms:

1. Whenever possible, *Avoid Medical Jargon*: It is important to note that there are times when medical jargon cannot be avoided. In those cases, one should be sure to define the medical term in a way that is easy for the patient or parent to understand.
2. Give the *Need-to-Know* important information up front: Medical handouts commonly start with disease pathophysiology and then move on to treatment and what to be on the alert for, the latter of which is what the patient really needs to know. Even when the treatment and symptoms to watch for are written in an easily understood prose, if they come after the dense information on pathophysiology, parents may stop reading before they get to the important information. Putting important information first ensures both that patients read it but and that they can have an easy place of reference if they have questions later [21].

3. Use Reading Level Eighth Grade of Below: The length of words and sentences determines reading levels in written information. The average reading level of a adults in the United States is below high school, however, medical handouts are often written at a tenth grade or higher reading level. Thus, all handouts in this resource were written at or below the eighth grade reading level.
4. User-Friendly layout with generous use of white space, large font, and pictures.

The American Academy of Pediatrics "Plain Language Pediatrics: Health Strategies and Communication Resources for Common Pediatric Topics" by Mary Ann Abrams, MD, MPH, FAAP and Benard P. Dreyer, MD, FAAP [21] is available for online purchase which provides access to the handouts themselves.

Many studies have confirmed patient satisfaction and ease of use of materials written in plain language. One study's objectives were to determine the health literacy skills of parents attending a pediatric surgery outpatient clinic and to describe parent satisfaction with plain-language materials. The authors found that the health literacy level of most patients was adequate; however, regardless of the parent's health literacy, there was overall satisfaction with the plain-language material. Satisfaction was measured using a survey questioning how easy the material was to read and understand, how informative it was, and how helpful it was [23]. Another study done in Australia interviewed parents after their children were discharged from the hospital. Specifically, they wanted to identify the parents' needs for information concerning their child's care following his or her discharge from hospital, and whether these needs were being met. Families reported that both verbal and written information were helpful but many received only verbal information. For those who did receive written information, some thought it was adequate, whereas others did not. Specifically, families thought that discharge summaries appeared unhelpful to parents, frequently because of the language used. Participants in both studies highlighted the need for discharge information to be provided in 'user-friendly' language [24]. They also sought individualized discharge information about their child's illness that included what to watch and expect after discharge [21, 24].

In summary, using plain language on medical forms can help families better understand the care they are receiving and potentially make health care more accessible to all people, regardless of their health literacy. Remember all of the steps in which a patient and his/her family encounter written materials throughout the process of seeing a physician? Now imagine if all of those written materials used plain language. How much easier would it be for a family to navigate the healthcare system and understand written information?

References

1. http://www.merriam-webster.com/dictionary/shame. Accessed 22 Feb 2016.
2. Baker DW, Parker RM, Williams MV, et al. The health care experience of patients with low literacy. Arch Fam Med. 1996;5(6):329–34.

3. Parikh NS, Parker RM, Nurss JR, et al. Shame and health literacy: the unspoken connection. Patient Educ Couns. 1996;27(1):33–9.
4. Wilson M. Readability and patient education materials used for low-income populations. Clin Nurse Spec. 2009;23(1):33–40.
5. D'Alessandro DM, Kingsley P, Johnson-West J. The readability of pediatric patient education materials on the World Wide Web. Arch Pediatr Adolesc Med. 2001;155(7):807–12.
6. Kirsch I, Jungeblut A, Jenkins L, et al. Adult literacy in America: a first look at the results of the National Adult Literacy Survey. Washington: National Center for Education Statistics, US Department of Education; 1993.
7. https://nces.ed.gov/pubs93/93275.pdf. Accessed 5 Feb 2016.
8. Weiss BD. Health literacy: a manual for clinicians. Chicago: American Medical Association Foundation and American Medical Association; 2003.
9. Nouri SS, Rudd RE. Health literacy in the "oral exchange": an important element of patient-provider communication. Patient Educ Couns. 2015;98(5):565–71.
10. Howe CJ, Cipher DJ, LeFlore J, et al. Parent health literacy and communication with diabetes educators in a pediatric diabetes clinic: a mixed methods approach. J Health Commun. 2015;20(Suppl 2):50–9.
11. Otal D, Wizowski L, Pemberton J, et al. Parent health literacy and satisfaction with plain language education materials in a pediatric surgery outpatient clinic: a pilot study. J Pediatr Surg. 2012;47(5):964–9.
12. Davis TC, Williams MV, Marin E, et al. Health literacy and cancer communication. CA Cancer J Clin. 2002;52(3):134–49.
13. Williams MV, Davis T, Parker RM, et al. The role of health literacy in patient-physician communication. Fam Med. 2002;34(5):383–9.
14. Mayeaux Jr EJ, Murphy PW, Arnold C, et al. Improving patient education for patients with low literacy skills. Am Fam Physician. 1996;53(1):205–11.
15. http://health.gov/communication/literacy/issuebrief/#adults. Accessed 24 Feb 2016.
16. http://www.plainlanguage.gov/plLaw/law/agency_pl_page.cfm. Accessed 24 Feb 2016.
17. World Bank. Adult learning and retention: factors and strategies. The learning pyramid. n.d. worldbank.org/DEVMARKETPLACE/Resources/Handout_TheLearningPyramid.pdf. Accessed 29 Feb 2016.
18. Langewitz W, Benz M, Keller A, et al. Spontaneous talking time at start of consultation in outpatient clinic: cohort study. BMJ. 2002;325:682–3.
19. Blau JN. Time to let the patient speak. BMJ. 1989;298:39.
20. Marvel MK, Epstein RM, Flowers K, Beckman HB. Soliciting the patient's agenda: have we improved? JAMA. 1999;281:283–7.
21. Keatinge DR, Stevenson K, Fitzgerald M. Parents' perceptions and needs of children's hospital discharge information. Int J Nurs Pract. 2009;15:341–7.
22. Plain language: what is plain language? Plainlanguage.gov. N.p. 2016 Web 25 Apr 2016.
23. Abrams MA, Dreyer BP, editors. Plain language pediatrics: health literacy strategies and communication resources for common pediatric topics. Illinois: American Academy of Pediatrics; 2009.
24. Otala D, Wizowskic L, Pembertona J, et al. Parent health literacy and satisfaction with plain language education materials in a pediatric surgery outpatient clinic: a pilot study. J Pediatr Surg. 2012;47:964–9.

Chapter 6
Health Literacy and Medical Education

Teri Turner

> *"What I hear, I forget. What I hear and see, I remember a little.*
> *What I hear, see and ask questions about or discuss with someone*
> *else, I begin to understand. What I hear, see, discuss, and do, I*
> *acquire knowledge and skill. What I teach to another I master."*
>
> —Mel Silberman 1942–2010 (Professor Emeritus at Temple
> University and a pioneer in the field of educational psychology
> and training)

The goal of this chapter is to provide an overview of the state of health literacy education in the health care professions and to provide resources that will be useful to individuals who are interested in personal development or would like to facilitate improvement in the systems in which care is delivered on a daily basis. Core competencies for effective communication between patient and provider are discussed first, followed by a review of strategies that have been used to change health care provider's behaviors and the outcomes of these efforts. A brief discussion of the science of learning is included to demonstrate how educational gaps can be filled using evidence-based strategies.

Providers' Communication Role to Enhance Patients' Adherence

"Drugs don't work in patients who don't take them."—C. Everett Koop 1916–2013
(13th Surgeon General of the United States)

Developing successful training programs requires identifying and implementing a conceptual model. One well established model is Ley's model on effective communication in practice (see Fig. 6.1) [1, 2].

T. Turner, MD, MPH, Med (✉)
Department of Pediatrics, Baylor College of Medicine, Texas Children's Hospital,
6621 Fannin Street, Clinical Care Center, Suite 1540.00, Houston, TX 77030-2399, USA
e-mail: turner@bcm.ed

© The Editor(s) and The Author(s) 2017   57
R.A. Connelly, T. Turner (eds.), *Health Literacy and Child Health Outcomes*,
SpringerBriefs in Public Health, DOI 10.1007/978-3-319-50799-6_6

Fig. 6.1 Overview of
Ley's model on the
interactions between
patient-related factors and
therapy adherence [1, 2]

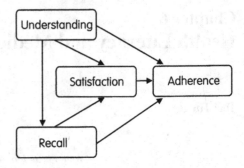

Within this framework, Ley stresses three key components that lead to patient adherence; understanding, recall, and satisfaction with the information provided [1]. A patient's non-adherence often is not a conscious choice but a failure of communication by the health care provider in one or more of these three areas. Hence, developing effective communication training programs that optimize patient outcomes will require addressing each of these areas individually.

In a national random survey of non-retired members of the American Academy of Pediatrics, almost all respondents (99%) reported using every day plain language when communicating with patients and their families [3]. However, actual practice of these behaviors in the clinical setting is likely much lower. Indeed, 81% of these same respondents stated they were aware of a time in the last 12 months in which a patient had not understood information that had been delivered to him or her [3]. Among a sample of pediatric residents, Farrell et al. reported a high instance of medical jargon, with rare explanations of these terms being used during parental counseling session about newborn screening results [4]. Maniaci et al. surveyed both patients and physicians about their perceptions of communication during the same clinical encounter. Compared to physicians, patients reported poorer perceptions of communication for the basic strategies of speaking slowly (18% lower) and using words that can be easily understood (32% lower) [5]. It is ultimately the health care provider's responsibility to ensure a patients' understanding. As stated so eloquently by George Bernard Shaw (1856–1950), *"The single biggest problem in communication is the illusion that it has taken place."* To be effective, training programs must first target this breakdown between what providers think they are communicating and the patient's actual experience.

Metaphorically, how human beings process information has been likened to a computer processing system; information is received, stored in memory and then retrieved as needed [6]. Receiving information that is understandable is the first step in the pathway to patient adherence. As much as 56% of information given to patients during a medical visit is forgotten shortly after the patient leaves the physician's office [7]. Several factors are related to retention or loss of information. For example, the greater the amount and complexity of information presented, the higher the likelihood it will be forgotten [2]. Kessels describes other factors, including older age of the patient/parent and one's emotional state that can impact memory [2]. With regard to the latter, Kessels notes that attention narrowing is particularly relevant in clinical care. For example when a parent hears the word "cancer" as a diagnosis for his or her child, other information that is delivered after this emotionally laden word, likely will not be remembered (i.e. attention narrowing). One also has to be able to focus on the information provided. For example, if a parent is trying to attend to several tasks such as soothing a crying child or monitoring a child's behavior, he or she will have difficulty not only listening and understanding the message that was conveyed but remembering later [8]. Based on research performed on human memory, individuals are also more likely to remember information that is given first, a phenomenon known as the 'primary effect' [2]. These types of advanced skills have a huge impact on patient outcomes but seldom are taught in health literacy training programs.

Further, information must be perceived as being important if it is to be understood, recalled, and acted upon. Studies conducted on trust in pediatric critical care settings demonstrate that most parents consider communication to be integral to building trust in the PICU [9]. Studies have found that African-Americans report lower feelings of trust in medical providers compared with Caucasians [10]. Minority parents, compared to nonminority parents, also report more frequently that doctors do not listen to their concerns [9, 10]. We found similar findings related to listening skills, trust, and shared decision-making among resident providers in the neonatal intensive care unit [11]. All parents, regardless of race and ethnicity, valued the following communication characteristics: honest, inclusive, compassionate, clear and comprehensive, and coordinated (what DeLemos et al. has called the "HICCC" mnemonic) [9].

Families are also more likely to trust information that comes from health care providers whom they perceive are most like them or whom they have known over a longer period of time [10, 12–15]. Satisfaction with the process of care can also impact trust. The physician's expertise in communication may not matter if the patients' prior health care experience was poor.

We have chosen to highlight these key components because they are not always implicitly included in training programs. Ley's theory of patient compliance provides a conceptual framework for enhancing the effectiveness of communication training: all three components—understanding, recall, and satisfaction—must be included if we as a health care team want to optimize patient adherence and outcomes [1].

Prevalence of Health Literacy Training

Coleman et al. surveyed 61 U.S. schools of allopathic medicine and found that 72% had formal curriculum on health literacy, which varied considerably by institution. The time spent on health literacy education ranged from 0 to 8 or more hours, with a median of 3 h [16]. Among those institutions with a required curriculum, most of the teaching occurred in the first 2 years of medical school training. Another study examined formal teaching in community-based internal medicine residency programs [17]. Of the 90 programs surveyed, one third participated. Eighty percent of all responding programs reported spending 3 or more hours on communication training. However, fewer than half of the respondents (43%) reported teaching health literacy as part of the residency curriculum. A similar study was conducted assessing health literacy teaching within U.S. family medicine programs [18]. Of the 444 programs surveyed, 138 responded (31%). Similar to the study in internal medicine, 42% of programs reported teaching health literacy as part of the required curriculum. The total hours of instruction ranged from 2 to 5 h, and most of the teaching occurred in the first year of post-graduate training. Interestingly, approximately two thirds of the respondents reported that resident physicians entering their programs had not been adequately trained in health literacy principles during medical school. The absence of a faculty member who was considered an authority in health literacy was strongly associated with the lack of residency training in this study.

Toronto undertook a literature review to examine health literacy education in health profession schools [19]. Five of the nine studies meeting inclusion criteria included pharmacy students, three included nursing students, and the ninth included internal medicine residents. No studies identified a longitudinal health literacy curriculum spanning the entire length of training nor did any discuss interprofessional learning. Only one study, reported conducting a formal needs assessment to determine learners baseline skills [20]. Most of the articles described a single class session, usually taught in the second or third year of entry-level health professional students' training. Conspicuously absent is any literature on required training for those who have completed formal health education professional training. However, the Accreditation Council of Continuing Medical Education (ACCME) has included, in its proposed new standards for excellence, communication training and evaluation of these skills [21]. The ACCME has also proposed having patients and families on continuing medical education planning committees.

Educational Competencies for Health Literacy Training

Coleman et al. conducted a consensus study using a modified Delphi method to identify health literacy educational competencies and target behaviors relevant to the training of all health care professionals [22]. Twenty-three experts in health profession education representing 11 of the 15 organizations belonging to the Federation of Associations of Schools of the Health Professions took part in this study. Consensus was reached on 62 educational competencies and 32 health literacy practices. However, because of methodological issues, the authors were not able to prioritize or rank-order these recommendations. The 62 educational competencies are divided into the domains of knowledge, attitudes, and skills. As the authors noted, there may also be significant overlap with other health communication constructs such as cross-cultural communication, general interviewing skills, motivational interviewing and shared decision making. This study does, however, provide an excellent starting point for health profession educators as they embark on developing their own training programs.

Table 6.1 Healthy People 2020 health communication objectives [27]

Increase the proportion of persons who report that their health care providers ALWAYS
1. Gave them easy-to-understand instructions about what to do to take care of their illness or health condition (HC/HIT-1.1—target 70.1%)
2. Asked them to describe how they will follow instructions (HC/HIT-1.2—target 26.9%)
3. Offered help in filling out a form (HC/HIT-1.3—target 16.3%)
4. Listened carefully to them (HC/HIT-2.1—target 65%)
5. Explained things so they could understand them (HC/HIT-2.2—target 66%)
6. Showed respect for what they had to say (HC/HIT-2.3—target 68.2%)
7. Spent enough time with them (HC/HIT-2.4—target 54%)
8. Involved them in decisions about their health care as much as they wanted (HC/HIT-3—target 56.8%)

HC/HIT Health Communication and Health Information Technology

The Association of American Medical Colleges has created recommendations for clinical skills curricula for undergraduate medical education in an effort to establish a national consensus regarding preclerkship clinical skills learning and outcomes. This task force recommended several competency goals and skill objectives to be obtained by the end of the preclerkship period in the domain of Patient Engagement and Communication Skill [23]. These skills include using plain language, effectively eliciting questions from the patient, and properly including and using an interpreter. The Accreditation Council of Graduate Medical Education also emphasizes communication skills in general within the domain of Interpersonal and Communication Skills [24]. Several specialties, including pediatrics, include specific competencies related to general communication skills that include the importance of "mitigating barriers to communication" in patient care [25]. This would include communicating with family members who have limited health literacy skills.

In 2015, the Advisory Committee on Training in Primary Care Medicine and Dentistry recommended in their report on health literacy and patient engagement that "skills to address health literacy be incorporated into all health professions activities..." [26]. They did not, however, provide specific information on what skills should be included. Additionally, seven objectives of Health People 2020 specifically focus on improving health care providers' communication skills (see Table 6.1) [27].

Curricular Content

In the health literacy content reported in the literature, marked variability exists concerning the essential components to teach. Of the 44 medical schools surveyed by Coleman et al., almost all respondents (95.5%) included plain language skills training for oral communication [16]. Eighty-four percent taught about the association between literacy and patient outcomes, and almost three-fourths (70.5%) included how to use a "teach back" or "show me" technique to check patients' understanding.

A similar percentage (70.5%) also included teaching on the prevalence of individuals with low health literacy skills. The two studies on post-graduate training found similar percentages of the same curricular content as well as a similar emphasis [17, 18]. Although percentages were not reported, Toronto et al., list these same topics in their literature review of health literacy education in health profession schools [19].

In 2003, the National Quality Forum listed the teach-back technique as a "top safety practice" and this recognition has been viewed as an endorsement to include this particular health literacy strategy as a top priority for health professions training [22]. McCleary-Jones conducted a systematic review of the literature on health literacy training in nursing education [28]. Based on the review, she provides thirteen recommendations for health literacy content topics, including items such as identifying individuals with limited health literacy, methods to enhance communication, plain language resources, best practice for written material and methods for verification of patient understanding, for nursing curricula. Training in communication skills, whether focused on health literacy specifically or not, will enhance the likelihood that information is understood. Thus, teachers should also seek out others who are currently teaching about communication in order to build upon existing curricular content for online resources (see Table 6.2).

Methods for Teaching Health Literacy Content

Numerous methods are effective in delivering content and are useful for developing curriculum. Far too often, curriculum designers depend on a more passive style of teaching such as lectures and didactics to deliver information. Studies in graduate medical education demonstrated that most family medicine and internal medicine programs utilized these methods (69% and 84%, respectively) [17, 18]. Evidence now indicates that active learning is more effective than is passive learning [29]. Armstrong and Parsa-Parsi describe how one can apply the principles of David Kolb's experiential learning theory to curriculum design in order to promote change in behavior [30, 31]. The authors incorporate the terminology used by McCarthy to describe four distinct areas that should be used in designing curriculum [30, 32].

These areas are labeled:

1. Activate prior knowledge (reflection on what the learner already knows)
2. What is the new knowledge? (enrich or expand on existing knowledge)
3. Try it out (practice)
4. Just do it (getting a commitment from the learner to change practice)

Just Health Action, a U.S.-based non-profit organization with the mission to reduce health inequities, has created a curricular framework using the principles described above for teaching health literacy within the context of social determinants of health [33]. Just Health Action uses Nutbeam's concept of 'critical health literacy' (one's understanding of the social determinants of health in conjunction with the skills to advocate for equality) as a framework for its curriculum, which

Table 6.2 Examples of resources for teaching about health literacy (Listed in alphabetical order)

Organization	Content	Methodology	Cost	CME or MOC credit	Location where materials can be found or purchased
Agency for Healthcare Research and Quality	Health Literacy Universal Precautions Toolkit, 2nd Edition	Online toolkit Print materials Videos Experiential activities	Free	No	http://www.ahrq.gov/ professionals/quality-patient-safety/quality-resources/tools/literacy-toolkit/healthlittoolkit2.html
Always Use Teach Back (UnityPoint Health, Picker Institute, Des Moines University, Health Literacy Iowa)	Always Use Teach Back toolkit	Online toolkit Videos Interactive module	Free	No	http://www.teachbacktraining.org/
American Academy of Pediatrics: Health Literacy Strategies to Enhance Communication	1. Health Literacy and Its Impact on Patient Care 2. Bridging the Communication Gap 3. Changing My Practice Environment	Online module includes case studies, videos, knowledge assessment questions and on-screen didactics	Non-Member: $48 AAP Member: $40 Resident Member: FREE	2 h CME credit	http://shop.aap.org/ Health-Literacy-Strategies-to-Enhance-Communication
American Board of Pediatrics	Improve Health Literacy Performance Improvement Module	Online module and Quality Improvement Project	Free for ABP diplomats	MOC and CME credit	https://www.abp.org/
American Medical Association Foundation: Health Literacy and Patient Safety: Help Patients Understand—Manual for Clinicians, 2nd edition	A 56 page overview of health literacy created in 2007	Print materials	Free download on some websites	No	Use web based search engine to locate the monograph http://med.fsu.edu/userFiles/file/ahec_health_clinicians_manual.pdf

(continued)

Table 6.2 (continued)

Organization	Content	Methodology	Cost	CME or MOC credit	Location where materials can be found or purchased
American Medical Association Foundation: Health Literacy and Patient Safety: Help Patients Understand: Reducing the Risk by Designing a Safer, Shame-Free Health Care Environment	This monograph also produced in 2007 explores how ineffective communication and low health literacy combine to affect patient safety, provides tools to decrease communication-related adverse events at a system wide level, and helps physicians initiate changes toward a safer and shame-free practice environment	Print materials	Free download on some websites	No	Use web based search engine to locate the monograph https://dshs.texas.gov/IDCU/health/infection_control/hai/hl_monograph.doc
Centers for Disease Control and Prevention (CDC) Health Literacy for Public Health Professionals	1. Health Literacy for Public Health Professionals 2. Writing for the Public 3. Using Numbers and Explaining Risk 4. Creating Easier to Understand Lists, Charts, and Graphs 5. Speaking with the Public	5 online modules includes case studies, videos, knowledge assessment questions and on-screen didactics	Free	1.25 CME for module 1 only	http://www.cdc.gov/healthliteracy/gettraining.html
MedEDPORTAL	Various training materials including "Health Literacy for Clerkship Students"	PowerPoint, cases, videos	Free	No	www.mededportal.org

Minnesota Health Literacy Partnership	1. Health Literacy 101 2. Health Numeracy 3. Teachback	PowerPoint presentations, speakers notes, videos, activities, knowledge assessments	Free	No	http://healthliteracymn.org/resources/presentations-and-training
The Ohio State University AHEC Health Literacy Distance Education Modules	12 different modules (~ 1 h in length) spanning written and oral communication skills	Web based learning modules	$20 one time registration fee and $15 per module	No	https://healthliteracy.osu.edu/

consists of four components: knowledge, 'compass,' skills (including tools), and action [34]. A unique aspect is their inclusion of 'compass' or experiential activities designed to help students "find their own direction as social change agents" at both the individual and community levels [33]. Mogford et al. describes the goal of 'compass' to "motivate students to advocate for health equity in a manner that suits their individual lifestyle and skill set." This section is further divided into four parts that facilitate this goal: "unpacking advocacy," "find your passion," "vision and goals," and "fuel your fire." The outcomes of this curriculum are not simply to improve health literacy knowledge and skills but also to elicit community-wide activism focused on decreasing health-care inequities. As the field of pediatrics focuses on the effects of poverty on the health and well-being of children, this framework can help curriculum developers design learning activities to teach health literacy within the construct of advocating on the social determinants of health.

Table 6.3 contains examples from the literature of techniques that have been used in various health literacy curricula across the educational spectrum. Coleman published a literature review in 2013, which includes findings from several implemented curricula [35]. Overviews of teaching methods can also be found either in review articles or descriptions of curricula [19, 20, 28, 33, 36–40]. Regardless of the method chosen, having participation by patients, patient's families or lay community health promotors can be a powerful tool for teaching [41]. This can be accomplished through the use of patient panels, videotaped patient narratives, or in simulated patient encounters.

Table 6.3 Teaching methods by Kolb experiential learning theory content area

Activate prior knowledge	New knowledge	Try it out	Just do it
• Written or verbal reflections on past experiences with low-health literacy patients • Patients telling about their health care experiences • Pre-tests of knowledge • Helping patients navigate the health care system (simulated or real encounters)	• Lectures/didactics • Assigned readings • Online training • Podcasts/Vodcasts • Watching a videotaped patient encounter followed by discussion • Case studies	• Role-playing • Standardized/ simulated patient encounters • Feedback following clinical encounters • Evaluating written (or printed) patient education materials, including assessing the material for reading level • Complete health literacy assessments on volunteers	• Action plans • Applied learning activities (out of 'class' assignments or activities to apply what has been learned in one's own environment) • Service learning projects

Educational Principles

Evidence for effective teaching strategies has increased over the past two decades. In particular, there is data now emerging on how the neurobiology of learning impacts medical education [42, 43]. Learning often requires multiple exposures to educational interventions before being incorporated into one's clinical practice. Competence in performing a skill requires deliberate practice and feedback [44, 45]. These skills fade quickly if not reinforced and/or regularly practiced [46].

Material learned is retained longer and efficiency of this learning is enhanced by the use of spaced repetition and practice [47–50]. Table 6.4 outlines twelve tips gleaned from the medical education literature to facilitate the creation of a health literacy curriculum using evidence-based practices.

Table 6.4 Twelve tips for creating a health literacy curriculum

1. Use a logical systematic approach such as Curriculum Development for Medical Education: A Six-Step Approach by Thomas et al. [55]
2. Conduct a needs assessment that includes both the learner's and patient's voices as stakeholders in the outcome of the curriculum
3. When deciding on goals and objectives, begin by using the competencies and practices described by Coleman et al. as a starting point and menu of options [22]
4. Experiential learning is crucial to an effective training session. David Kolb's four stage model provides an excellent framework and consists of
(a) Reflecting on experience
(b) Assimilating and conceptualizing information
(c) Experimenting and practicing
(d) Planning for application [31, 32]
5. Active learning is more effective than is passive learning. Use several active learning strategies such as discussions, video review, and large group brainstorming sessions in delivering the curriculum rather than relying heavily on passive learning through didactic teaching
6. What we think we know already (or a skill we think we do well) is the greatest barrier to learning. Incorporate exercises that create cognitive dissonance (i.e., challenges to these assumptions) to enhance learning
7. Make learning authentic. Integrate health literacy training into the clinical context instead of teaching it in isolation. One of the best methods is to use actual case examples encountered in clinical practice
8. Incorporate ample time to practice health literacy skills and receive feedback using small group role play activities, simulated patient encounters, or standardized patients
9. Assess whether learning has occurred during training sessions and evaluate transfer of skills to clinical practice after the curriculum is completed. The ways in which trainees are assessed and evaluated powerfully affects the way in which they learn
10. Mastering a skill or learning a body of knowledge takes time and cannot be accomplished in one sitting. Refresher training is needed to maintain competence. Use the 'spacing effect' (deliver and repeat information over time) to enhance what is retained [47–50]
11. Whenever possible provide credit for professional development such as hours of continuous medical education or maintenance of certification credit. Even certificates of competence or mastery provide an incentive for learning
12. Don't "reinvent the wheel." Several curricular components (case studies, videos, exercises, etc.) are already developed. Contact the authors of studies of health literacy training programs to see if they would be willing to share their materials which can serve as a great starting point for your own curriculum

Assessment

"I taught Stripe (sic my dog) how to whistle." "I don't hear him whistling."
"I said I taught him, I didn't say he learned it." —From the comic strip "Tiger" by Bud
Blake (1918–2005) King Features Syndicate.

Without assessment, we do not know whether our trainees have learned. It is also often said that "it is what you inspect, not what you expect, that learners see as important." The first statement is an example of assessment *of* learning, the latter, assessment *for* learning. Both methods are beneficial when developing curricula, particular for health literacy. In the study of medical school curriculum, Coleman and Appy found that almost 57% of respondents assessed students using some type of simulated or standardized observation of a clinical encounter specifically designed for testing purposes [16]. Almost half used clinical observation in the workplace. A little more than a third (38.6%) used a written examination to assess learning outcomes. Among graduate medical education programs, direct observation was the most commonly used tool [17, 18]. Other techniques included patient satisfaction questionnaires, standardized encounters, and multisource (aka 360°) feedback. Written examinations were used least frequently.

In considering what to examine, a common delineation among evaluators, is to divide assessment into three domains: knowledge, attitude, and skill. Table 6.5 lists different types of assessment methods one could use when assessing each of these three domains. In the systematic review, Toronto et al., found several studies that assessed a combination of these three areas [19]. Just over three fourths (77.8%) of the studies administered pre- and post-tests to assess knowledge acquisition and two thirds assessed attitudes. Only one study assessed a change in skills. When selecting tools for assessment, curriculum designers should use several assessment methods and select the best strategy to match one's goals and objectives (i.e., the desired outcomes).

During the past several years, a shift to competency-based education and assessment in the health professions has occurred, particularly in graduate medical education [51]. Miller proposed a framework consisting of four stages in which an individual progresses from knowledge acquisition to performance in the clinical setting [52].

Table 6.5 Types of assessment by domain

Knowledge	Attitude	Skills
Knows what	*Knows why*	*Knows how*
• Written examinations • Chart reviews • Case discussions • Oral examinations • Presentations	• Global rating scales • Self-assessment surveys • Critical incident analysis • Reflection exercises • Multisource feedback based on clinical observations	• Direct observation and feedback • Videotape reviews • Objective Structured Clinical Examination (OSCE) or Clinical Performance Exam (CPX) • Checklists • Chart review • Projects

These stages are "knows, knows how, shows how (i.e., competence) and does (i.e., performance)." The ultimate way to assess a trainee's application of health literacy skills in the clinical environment is to ask his or her patients. It's not enough to be able to show that you can use plain language, rather we must assess whether the patient understood what his or her doctor said. Regardless of the tool used, always look at the way you assess and ask yourself—"How will this benefit my learners?"

Program Evaluation: Do Health Literacy Curricula Have an Impact on the Patient and Society?

Most studies describe the impact of health literacy curricula on participants. For example, the authors of three systematic reviews of the literature describe several studies which demonstrated a change in participant knowledge but fewer studies which demonstrated a change in health literacy attitudes or skills [19, 28, 35]. Connelly et al. reported an increase in physician self-reported use of health literacy communication techniques from a 3 h workshop with community practitioners [37]. Similarly, Clark et al. reported that pediatricians who received training on communicating with patients and families with asthma were rated by parents as better communicators on all performance measures in comparison to physicians in the control group [53]. When assessing the impact on patient outcomes or the society, far less is known. Mogford et al. showed an increase "empowerment to act on the social determinants of health" at the individual, community and organizational level among participants in their curriculum [33]. Coleman points out that although training in health literacy is associated with positive educational outcomes, the findings from these individual studies cannot be generalized due to a lack of consistent or validated outcome measures [35]. Yin et al. has proposed a conceptual framework which describe how Health Literacy is a potential "Educationally Sensitive Patient Outcome or ESPO" [54]. They propose that education aimed to improve physician's use of health literacy strategies, to 'activate the patient in their own self-care' taking into account the system in which this care is being delivered, leads to meaningful, patient outcomes. These authors stress, as does Coleman, that we must begin to explore and measures these links [35, 54].

Summary

In this chapter, we have provided an overview of health literacy education outlining the discussion within the context of a curriculum framework. Patient adherence is a complex interplay of understanding, recall, and satisfaction with the information provided. As teachers, we must include these components in our educational activities if we want to improve patient adherence. There is a paucity of data on what teaching methods are most effective in transferring health literacy skills to the clinical environment. We also know that teaching, in and of itself, will not guarantee that our students have learned. We do have, however, several examples of curricula to build upon when designing our own learning experiences. We have also listed several examples of active learning techniques that have been shown to increase skills and engagement with patients and the community. Mastery of health literacy communication skills requires continuous practice and feedback. True efficacy as a physician is defined not only by what he or she knows but what the physician is able to get across to his or her patients. Pediatricians must not only know there is a problem, but also have the motivation and drive to change, gain knowledge and skills, implement changes, measure the results of those changes and reflect on the outcomes in order to improve the quality of care to all patients.

References

1. Ley P. Communicating with patients: improving communication, satisfaction and compliance. London: Croom Helm; 1988.
2. Kessels RP. Patients' memory for medical information. J R Soc Med. 2003;96(5):219–22.
3. Turner T, Cull WL, Bayldon B, et al. Pediatricians and health literacy: descriptive results from a national survey. Pediatrics. 2009;124(Suppl 3):S299–305.
4. Farrell M, Deuster L, Donovan J, Christopher S. Pediatric residents' use of jargon during counseling about newborn genetic screening results. Pediatrics. 2008;122(2):243–9.
5. Maniaci MJ, Heckman MG, Dawson NL. Physician versus patient perception of physician hospital discharge communication: a preliminary study. Open J Intern Med. 2014;4(04):101.
6. Schunk DH. Learning theories: an educational perspective. 6th ed. Boston: Pearson; 2012.
7. Ley P, Spelman MS. Communications in an out-patient setting. Br J Soc Clin Psychol. 1965;4(2):114–6.
8. Abrams MA, Dreyer BP. American Academy of Pediatrics. Plain language pediatrics: health literacy strategies and communication resources for common pediatric topics. Elk Grove: American Academy of Pediatrics; 2009.
9. DeLemos D, Chen M, Romer A, et al. Building trust through communication in the intensive care unit: HICCC. Pediatr Crit Care Med. 2010;11(3):378–84.
10. Doescher MP, Saver BG, Franks P, Fiscella K. Racial and ethnic disparities in perceptions of physician style and trust. Arch Fam Med. 2000;9(10):1156–63.
11. Mack T, Turner T, Profit J, Raphael J. Parental assessment of resident physician cultural competence in the Neonatal Intensive Care Unit [abstract]. Boston: Pediatric Academic Societies; 2012: E-PAS2012:3819.233.
12. Street Jr RL, O'Malley KJ, Cooper LA, Haidet P. Understanding concordance in patient-physician relationships: personal and ethnic dimensions of shared identity. Ann Fam Med. 2008;6(3):198–205.
13. Wissow LS, Brown JD, Krupnick J. Therapeutic alliance in pediatric primary care: preliminary evidence for a relationship with physician communication style and mothers' satisfaction. J Dev Behav Pediatr. 2010;31(2):83–91.
14. Christakis DA, Mell L, Koepsell TD, Zimmerman FJ, Connell FA. Association of lower continuity of care with greater risk of emergency department use and hospitalization in children. Pediatrics. 2001;107(3):524–9.
15. Love MM, Mainous III AG, Talbert JC, Hager GL. Continuity of care and the physician-patient relationship: the importance of continuity for adult patients with asthma. J Fam Pract. 2000;49(11):998–1004.

16. Coleman CA, Appy S. Health literacy teaching in US medical schools, 2010. Fam Med. 2012;44(7):504–7.
17. Ali NK. Are we training residents to communicate with low health literacy patients? J Community Hosp Intern Med Perspect. 2012;2(4).
18. Coleman CA, Nguyen NT, Garvin R, Sou C, Carney PA. Health literacy teaching in U.S. family medicine residency programs: a national survey. J Health Commun. 2016;21(Suppl 1):51–7.
19. Toronto CE, Weatherford B. Health literacy education in health professions schools: an integrative review. J Nurs Educ. 2015;54(12):669–76.
20. Green JA, Gonzaga AM, Cohen ED, Spagnoletti CL. Addressing health literacy through clear health communication: a training program for internal medicine residents. Patient Educ Couns. 2014;95(1):76–82.
21. Accreditation Council for Continuing Medical Education (ACCME). Proposal for new criteria for accreditation with commendation. http://www.accme.org/requirements/accreditation-requirements-cme-providers/proposal-new-criteria-accreditation-commendation. Accessed 11 June 2016.
22. Coleman CA, Hudson S, Maine LL. Health literacy practices and educational competencies for health professionals: a consensus study. J Health Commun. 2013;18(Suppl 1):82–102.
23. Association of American Medical Colleges (AAMC). Core entrustable professional activities for entering residency. Faculty and learners guide. 2014. http://members.aamc.org/eweb/upload/Core%20EPA%20Faculty%20and%20Learner%20Guide.pdf. Accessed 10 June 2016.
24. Batalden P, Leach D, Swing S, Dreyfus H, Dreyfus S. General competencies and accreditation in graduate medical education. Health Aff (Project Hope). 2002;21(5):103–1.
25. Benson BJ. Domain of competence: interpersonal and communication skills. Acad Pediatr. 2014;14(2 Suppl):S55–65.
26. Advisory Committee on Training in Primary Care Medicine and Dentistry. Health literacy and patient engagement. Twelfth annual report to the secretary of the United States Department of Health and Human Services and the Congress of the United States. 2015. http://www.hrsa.gov/advisorycommittees/bhpradvisory/actpcmd/Reports/twelfthreport.pdf. Accessed 11 June 2016.
27. Healthy People 2020 Framework: the vision, mission, and goals of Healthy People 2020. http://www.healthypeople.gov. Accessed 10 June 2016.
28. McCleary-Jones V. A systematic review of the literature on health literacy in nursing education. Nurse Educ. 2016;41(2):93–7.
29. Prince M. Does active learning work? A review of the research. J Eng Educ. 2004;93(3):223–31.
30. Armstrong E, Parsa-Parsi R. How can physicians' learning styles drive educational planning? Acad Med. 2005;80(7):680–4.
31. Kolb DA. Experiential learning: experience as the source of learning and development. 2nd ed. Englewood Cliffs: Prentice Hall; 2013.
32. McCarthy B, O'Neill-Blackwell J. Hold on, you lost me!: use learning styles to create training that sticks. Alexandria: ASTD Press; 2007.
33. Mogford E, Gould L, Devoght A. Teaching critical health literacy in the US as a means to action on the social determinants of health. Health Promot Int. 2011;26(1):4–13.
34. Nutbeam D. Health literacy as a public health goal: a challenge for contemporary health education and communication strategies into the 21st century. Health Promot Int. 2000;15(3):259–67.
35. Coleman C. Teaching health care professionals about health literacy: a review of the literature. Nurs Outlook. 2011;59(2):70–8.
36. Connelly RA, Turner TL, Tran XG, Giardino AP. Lessons learned from using health literacy strategies in a pilot communication skills program. Open Pediatr Med J. 2010;4:26–32.
37. Connelly RA, Tran XG, Xu L, Giardino AP, Turner TL. Increased use of health literacy strategies for communication by physicians. Health Behav Policy Rev. 2014;1(6):460–71.
38. Ha H, Lopez T. Developing health literacy knowledge and skills through case-based learning. Am J Pharm Educ. 2014;78(1):17.
39. Devraj R, Butler LM, Gupchup GV, Poirier TI. Active-learning strategies to develop health literacy knowledge and skills. Am J Pharm Educ. 2010;74(8):137.

40. Milford E, Morrison K, Teutsch C, et al. Out of the classroom and into the community: medical students consolidate learning about health literacy through collaboration with Head Start. BMC Med Educ. 2016;16(1):121.
41. Pagels P, Kindratt T, Arnold D, Brandt J, Woodfin G, Gimpel N. Training family medicine residents in effective communication skills while utilizing promotoras as standardized patients in OSCEs: a Health literacy curriculum. Int J Family Med. 2015;2015:129187.
42. Friedlander MJ, Andrews L, Armstrong EG, et al. What can medical education learn from the neurobiology of learning? Acad Med. 2011;86(4):415–20.
43. Mahan JD, Stein DS. Teaching adults-best practices that leverage the emerging understanding of the neurobiology of learning. Curr Probl Pediatr Adolesc Health Care. 2014;44(6):141–9.
44. Ericsson KA. Acquisition and maintenance of medical expertise: a perspective from the expert-performance approach with deliberate practice. Acad Med. 2015;90(11):1471–86.
45. McGaghie WC, Barsuk JH, Wayne DB. AM last page: mastery learning with deliberate practice in medical education. Acad Med. 2015;90(11):1575.
46. Pusic MV, Kessler D, Szyld D, Kalet A, Pecaric M, Boutis K. Experience curves as an organizing framework for deliberate practice in emergency medicine learning. Acad Emerg Med Off J Soc Acad Emerg Med. 2012;19(12):1476–80.
47. Kerfoot BP, Fu Y, Baker H, Connelly D, Ritchey ML, Genega EM. Online spaced education generates transfer and improves long-term retention of diagnostic skills: a randomized controlled trial. J Am Coll Surg. Sep 2010;211(3):331–7.e331.
48. Kerfoot BP. Adaptive spaced education improves learning efficiency: a randomized controlled trial. J Urol. 2010;183(2):678–81.
49. Kerfoot BP. Learning benefits of on-line spaced education persist for 2 years. J Urol. 2009;181(6):2671–3.
50. Kerfoot BP, DeWolf WC, Masser BA, Church PA, Federman DD. Spaced education improves the retention of clinical knowledge by medical students: a randomised controlled trial. Med Educ. 2007;41(1):23–31.
51. Nasca TJ, Philibert I, Brigham T, Flynn TC. The next GME accreditation system--rationale and benefits. New Engl JMed. 2012;366(11):1051–6.
52. Miller GE. The assessment of clinical skills/competence/performance. Acad Med. 1990;65(9 Suppl):S63–7.
53. Clark NM, Gong M, Schork MA, et al. Impact of education for physicians on patient outcomes. Pediatrics. 1998;101(5):831–6.
54. Yin HS, Jay M, Maness L, Zabar S, Kalet A. Health literacy: an educationally sensitive patient outcome. J Gen Intern Med. 2015;30(9):1363–8.
55. Thomas PA, Kern DE, Hughes MT, Chen BY. Curriculum development for medical education: a six-step approach. 3rd ed. Baltimore: John Hopkins University Press; 2015.

Chapter 7
Health Literacy and Child Health Outcomes: Dissemination and Sustainability of Improvement Efforts and Policy Changes

Angelo P. Giardino

> *"All systems and organization are faced with the challenge of implementing new practices at one time or another, yet many of the innovations that are initially successful fail to become part of the habits and routines of the host organizations and communities. Why do some take root and flourish while others languish?"*
>
> —*Wiltsey-Stirman et al. (2012) [1]*

Taken as a whole, the previous six chapters make a strong case for (1) the problems associated with low patient and parental health literacy, (2) the prospects for improved health outcomes by addressing the health literacy skills of health care systems, as well as those of patients and/or their families, and (3) the best practices that have been designed and tested such as a "universal precautions approach" and techniques such as "teach back," "chunk and check" and "using plain language", that is avoiding medical jargon. But, these previous chapters also document the regretfully slow and lumbering progress we are making as a nation in terms of the state of health literacy skills and best practices for health communication, disseminating the best practices among health care providers, and sustaining these enhanced elements of health communication in the long term practice.

This lack of progress for sustaining and spreading innovations in the health care system is not isolated to the health literacy arena. Towards that point, looking at health care innovations across a spectrum of care processes, it has been reported that innovations are _not_ sustained in the range from 33 to 70% of the times, as measured by a number of different organizational design methods [2]. Colleagues from the United Kingdom refer to this elusive goal of sustained change as the "evaporation

A.P. Giardino, MD, MPH, PhD (✉)
Department of Pediatrics, Baylor College of Medicine, Texas Children's Hospital,
2450 Holcombe, Suite 34L Houston, TX 77021, USA
e-mail: giardino@bcm.edu

© The Editor(s) and The Author(s) 2017
R.A. Connelly, T. Turner (eds.), *Health Literacy and Child Health Outcomes*,
SpringerBriefs in Public Health, DOI 10.1007/978-3-319-50799-6_7

of innovation" as they seek to capture disappointing inability to maintain enhanced improvement on a team, throughout the organization or across an entire country [3].

As the quote that began this chapter asks, *"Why do some take root and flourish while others languish?"* In more simple plain language, one can't help but ask, "How can this be?" Clearly, defining the problem, in this case, low levels of health literacy and developing approaches and techniques to rectify that situation are not enough! We need a more robust approach to actually see sustained efforts directed at promoting higher levels of health literacy and more informed health care practice to be realized with the resulting improved outcomes that we all in health care desire.

Health Literacy has been described as 'a policy challenge for advancing high-quality health care' [4]. Over the past few years there have been several federal policy initiatives to improve outcomes associated with low health literacy, including the quality improvement aspects of the Patient Protection and Affordable Care Act of 2010, the Department of Health and Human Services' National Action Plan to Improve Health Literacy, and the Plain Writing Act of 2010 [5]. In a defining, seminal report, the Institute of Medicine (IOM) issued "Health Literacy: A Prescription to End Confusion" which outlined necessary areas of focus for us to collectively target interventions [6]. Prominent among the systems that need attention are the health care system, the education system, and our culture and societal views as well [6]. Table 7.1 below depicts the set of recommendations from the IOM report by themes [6].

Chao et al. call for a national agenda focusing on health literacy and health disparities as a critical component of all quality improvement efforts [7]. Reflecting on the health care system and its providers, there has been a call for more education as outlined in Chap. 6 of this monograph.

Table 7.1 Recommendations from: 'A Prescription to End Confusion' [6]

Recommendations
Theme: Definition and Measures of Health Literacy

2.1	The Department of Health and Human Services and other government and private funders should support research leading to the development of causal models explaining the relationships among health literacy, the education system, the health system, and relevant social and cultural systems
2.2	The Department of Health and Human Services and public and private funders should support the development, testing, and use of culturally appropriate new measures of health literacy. Such measures should be developed for large ongoing population surveys, such as the National Assessment of Adult Literacy Survey, Medical Expenditure Panel Survey, and Behavioral Risk Factor Surveillance System, and the Medicare Beneficiaries Survey, as well as for institutional accreditation and quality assessment activities such as those carried out by the Joint Commission on Accreditation of Healthcare Organizations and the National Committee for Quality Assurance. Initially, the National Institutes of Health should convene a national consensus conference to initiate the development of operational measures of health literacy which would include contextual measures

(continued)

Table 7.1 (continued)

Recommendations

Theme: Extent of Limited Health Literacy in USA

3.1	Given the compelling evidence noted above, funding for health literacy research is urgently needed. The Department of Health and Human Services, especially the National Institutes of Health, Agency for Healthcare Research and Quality, Health Resources and Services Administration, the Centers for Disease Control and Prevention, Department of Defense, Veterans Administration, and other public and private funding agencies should support multidisciplinary research on the extent, associations, and consequences of limited health literacy, including studies on health service utilization and expenditures

Theme: Culture and Society

4.1	Federal agencies responsible for addressing disparities should support the development of conceptual frameworks on the intersection of culture and health literacy to direct in-depth theoretical explorations and formulate the conceptual underpinnings that can guide interventions **4.1a** The National Institutes of Health should convene a consensus conference, including stakeholders, to develop methodology for the incorporation of health literacy improvement into approaches to health disparities **4.1b** The Office of Minority Health and Agency for Healthcare Research and Quality should develop measures of the relationships between culture, language, cultural competency, and health literacy to be used in studies of the relationship between health literacy and health outcomes
4.2	The Agency for Healthcare Research and Quality, the Centers for Disease Control and Prevention, the Indian Health Service, the Health Resources and Services Administration, and the Substance Abuse and Mental Health Services Administration should develop and test approaches to improve health communication that foster healing relationships across culturally diverse populations. This includes investigations that explore the effect of existing and innovative communication approaches on health behaviors, and studies that examine the impact of participatory action and empowerment research strategies for effective penetration of health information at the community level

Theme: Educational Systems

5.1	Accreditation requirements for all public and private educational institutions should require the implementation of the National Health Education Standards
5.2	Educators should take advantage of the opportunity provided by existing reading, writing, reading, oral language skills, and mathematics curricula to incorporate health-related tasks, materials, and examples into existing lesson plans
5.3	The Health Resources and Services Administration and the Centers for Disease Control and Prevention, in collaboration with the Department of Education, should fund demonstration projects in each state to attain the National Health Education Standards and to meet basic literacy requirements as they apply to health literacy
5.4	The Department of Education in association with the Department of Health and Human Services should convene task forces comprised of appropriate education, health, and public policy experts to delineate specific, feasible, and effective actions relevant agencies could take to improve health literacy through the nation's K-12 schools, 2-year and 4-year colleges and universities, and adult and vocational education
5.5	The National Science Foundation, the Department of Education, and the National Institute of Child Health and Human Development should fund research designed to assess the effectiveness of different models of combining health literacy with basic literacy and instruction. The Interagency Education Research Initiative, a federal partnership of these three agencies, should lead this effort to the fullest extent possible

(continued)

Table 7.1 (continued)

	Recommendations
5.6	Professional schools and professional continuing education programs in health and related fields, including medicine, dentistry, pharmacy, social work, anthropology, nursing, public health, and journalism, should incorporate health literacy into their curricula and areas of competence
	Theme: Health Systems
6.1	Health care systems, including private systems, Medicare, Medicaid, the Department of Defense, and the Veterans Administration should develop and support demonstration programs to establish the most effective approaches to reducing the negative effects of limited health literacy. To accomplish this, these organizations should: • Engage consumers in the development of health communications and infuse insights gained from them into health messages • Explore creative approaches to communicate health information using printed and electronic materials and media in appropriate and clear language. Messages must be appropriately translated and interpreted for diverse audiences • Establish methods for creating health information content in appropriate and clear language using relevant translations of health information • Include cultural and linguistic competency as an essential measure of quality of care
6.2	The Department of Health and Human Services should fund research to define the needed health literacy tasks and skills for each of the priority areas for improvement in health care quality. Funding priorities should include participatory research which engages the intended populations
6.3	Health literacy assessment should be a part of healthcare information systems and quality data collection. Public and private accreditation bodies, including Medicare, the National Committee for Quality Assurance, and the Joint Commission on Accreditation of Healthcare Organizations should clearly incorporate health literacy into their accreditation standards
6.4	The Department of Health and Human Services should take the lead in developing uniform standards for addressing health literacy in research applications. This includes addressing the appropriateness of research design and methods and the match among the readability of instruments, the literacy level, and the cultural and linguistic needs of study participants. In order to achieve meaningful research outcomes in all fields: • Investigators should involve patients (or subjects) in the research process to ensure that methods and instrumentation are valid and reliable and in a language easily understood • The National Institutes of Health should collaborate with appropriate federal agencies and institutional review boards to formulate the policies and criteria to ensure that appropriate consideration of literacy is an integral part of the approval of research involving human subjects • The National Institutes of Health should take literacy levels into account when considering informed consent in human subjects research. Institutional Review Boards should meet existing standards related to the readability of informed consent documents

Adapted from: Institute of Medicine (U.S.). Committee on Health Literacy & Nielsen-Bohlman, L. *Health literacy: A prescription to end confusion.* Washington, D.C.: National Academies Press. http://www.nationalacademies.org/hmd/Reports/2004/Health-Literacy-A-Prescription-to-End-Confusion.aspx p. 14–16 [6]

However, knowledge alone will not cause providers to change. True transformation requires converting knowledge into practice. Once gaps are identified, resources need to be made available to improve these skills. According to Schwartz and Axelrad, focusing specifically on health literacy and adherence, "...education is necessary but not sufficient" to promote better adherence and ultimately better health outcomes (p. 25) [8]. The research they review argues strongly for interventions that combine educational efforts with behavioral approaches to allow for skill building along with an increase in knowledge and understanding.

Citing Schwartz and Axelrad's summary of the literature with a specific focus on parental involvement in child health, we read [8]:

"1. Health literacy involves a complex set of skills that include reading, math (numeracy), multimedia, problem-solving and interpretive skills.
2. Health literacy is closely associated with general literacy, and with socioeconomic and cultural factors that are themselves related to literacy ...
3. Health literacy *"must be considered in terms of parents' or caregivers' health literacy as well as the children's own health literacy* (which is evolving as children grow, learn, and develop)"...
4. Low parent health literacy is associated with worse child health outcomes, especially for younger children.
5. Low health literacy among adolescent is associated with greater general risk-taking behavior but there is no evidence of an association with worse adherence.
6. Overall, low health literacy is associated with worse adherence, BUT
7. Interventions to improve health literacy have been shown to improve health knowledge but at best have weak and indirect effects on health *behavior*

... Education is an important component of interventions ... however ... interventions that combine educational with behavioral approaches had more potent effects on health outcomes ... than either type of approach alone..."

—*Schwartz and Axelrad (p. 25)* [8]

In this chapter we will examine several frameworks that can serve to inform our collective efforts at avoiding the "evaporation of innovation" that all too often short circuits our efforts to improve both the health systems sensitivity to low health literacy, as well as our patients' efforts to improve their own health literacy skills.

Health Literacy and Quality Improvement

The change process and quality improvement efforts directed at improving health literacy and ultimately at improving care and outcomes are essential and must be well designed, spread and sustained. And by understanding the milieu in which health care occurs, we are then best positioned to advocate for change a change and quality improvement process that will actually produce the improved different results we seek to achieve.

First, we will explore an influence model that looks at motivation and capacity for the desired change at different levels of action [9]. Next, we will move on to explore a model for describing "educationally sensitive outcomes" (ESPOs) as a means for operationalizing the health care systems training needs in the health literacy arena [9]. This measurement approach is essential since a generally accepted management principle states, "if you can't measure it, then you can't manage it." Then we will examine the Model for Improvement, a simple but elegant model that nearly universally forms the basis of good deal of quality improvement work in health care [10]. Finally, we will conclude with a suggested approach to sustainability and spread and relate this back to the IOM's recommendations for action in the health care system.

> *"...When it comes to changing the world, what most lack is not the courage to change things, but the skill to do so."*
>
> —*Influence Model by Patterson et al.* [9]

Patterson and colleagues focus on how to influence people in various settings to make changes needed to achieve a stated goal [9]. Their analysis shows that successful change efforts focus on implementing a few behavior changes that can drive a large amount of change in a given setting. They call these few high-impact changes or behaviors 'vital behaviors' [9].

The Influence Model for Change Processes

The first step in the influence model is to respond to two questions at the start of any change process:

1. The first question relates to the motivation to undertake the hard work to make the necessary change. The question is *"should we make the change"*—essentially, *"will it be worth it?"*
2. The second question relates to the ability to make the change. The question is *"can we make the change"*—essentially, *"can we do it?"*

If the answer to the first question is no, then there is no motivation to continue the change effort. But, if it is yes, then we progress to the second question about ability to make the change. If the answer to "can we make the change" is no, then some skill building at the outset is necessary prior to proceeding. If the answer to "can we make the change" is yes, or becomes yes after suitable skill building, then a detailed plan, modeled like a quality improvement effort should be pursued. For the changes that we should make, and ones that we have the capability to undertake, Patterson and colleagues then progress to describing the individual, social and structural aspects of influencing the motivation to make a change, as well as the individual, social and structural aspects of influencing the ability to make the changes [9].

This model seeks to establish a link between motivation for change (*"should we do do it?"*) and variables that relate to the ability to make a change ("can we do it") at the individual, social or institutional and social levels. Central to the influence model is moving beyond "telling" people what things to do differently and instead finding opportunities for those involved to "experience" (either actual or vicarious) the results that come from doing things differently. Table 7.2 shows a table where a

Table 7.2 Six sources of influence as applied to health literacy

	Individual	Social	Structural
Motivation: **"Should we do it?"**	Yes Nearly universal experience of clinicians that message sent is not always message received	Yes "more than 78 million persons, scored in either the Below Basic or Basic level" (National Assessment of Adult Literacy (NAAL), 2003)	Yes "Health Literacy: A Prescription to End Confusion" (Institute of Medicine (IOM), 2004)
Ability: **"Can we do it?"**	Yes "teach back," "chunk and check" and "using plain language", avoids medical jargon	Yes "...offer a plan to improve communication without increasing time by following the "universal precautions" principle of giving all parents brief, to-the-point, concrete and specific information focused what they need to know and do, and pointing out the benefits." (Terry C Davis, Ph.D.)	Yes "Health care systems, including private systems, Medicare, Medicaid, the Department of Defense, and the Veterans Administration should develop and support demonstration programs to establish the most effective approaches to reducing the negative effects of limited health literacy." (IOM, 2004)

leadership group could use to identify potential changes at the individual, social and structural levels.

The theoretical underpinning of this approach comes from Albert Bandura's work on social learning theory and his observation that our behaviors in a given setting are largely shaped by our observing the behaviors of those around us [10]. Essentially, we tend to learn less from what we are told to do and we tend to learn more from watching the behaviors of others around us. So, experiences along with knowledge are fundamental to promoting change. The most likely successful change efforts are likely to be those opportunities that offer both knowledge (i.e. didactics) and experiences (i.e. workshops, role plays, video clips). As a result, the influence model is hinged on opportunities to practice newly acquired skills around the few vital behaviors [9].

In Patterson and colleagues' words:

"Break tasks into discrete actions, set goals for each, practice within a low-risk environment, and build in recovery strategies ... Many of the vital behaviors required to solve profound and persistent problems demand advanced interpersonal problem-solving skills that can be mastered only through well-researched, deliberate practice." [9] (p. 135)

The influence model can be readily applied to motivating health care providers towards improving their communication practices by recognizing the predominance of low levels of health literacy among many of their patients.

First, in response to *"should we do it?"* there is a resounding yes based on the body of evidence summarized in the first six chapters of this monograph. Clearly it's "worth" doing on many levels as has been stated throughout. Second, in response to *"can we do it?"*—again, a resounding yes in that we can, in fact, do better in health care communication during the health encounter, by adopting a few vital behaviors such as using a universal precautions approach, using teach back, chunking and checking, and avoiding medical jargon.

Text Box 1: Texas Children's Health Plan Feasibility Pilot: *"Should We Do It?"*

Connelly, RA, Turner, TL, Tran, XG and Giardino, AP (2010). **Lessons Learned from Using Health
Literacy Strategies in a Pilot Communication Skills Program.** *The Open Pediatric Medicine Journal,* 2010, *4,* 26–32

Abstract	Summary of the Themes, Based on Participants' Responses
Introduction: Limited health literacy results in poorer health outcomes, however, effective communication can facilitate understanding. Communication skills programs could incorporate strategies to address communication gaps caused by poor health literacy	*Reasons for participating:* • Willingness to improve communication skills; learn something new/new ways to communicate with patients effectively • Participant's realization that there is a disconnect, miscommunication between patients and providers • Wanted to learn how to build up rapport with patients through communication, better communication • Learn ways to communicate better/reach out to challenging patients
Objectives: (1) to describe the effects of a pilot educational intervention on providers' knowledge and reported use of health literacy strategies; (2) to describe participants' reasons to participate and their opinions regarding the educational intervention's delivery and content	*Opinions regarding educational intervention* *Liked the most* • Interactive learning: interaction, small groups, active participation, role play exercise • New concept: there is a communication mismatch • Simple and practical advice on effective ways to communicate *Liked the least* • Time/Location: given on a Saturday morning, remote location • Not getting syllabus or materials for the workshop ahead of time • One participant reported she/he did not learn anything new, 'just basic things' participant felt already knew and did
Methodology: We conducted a quasi-experimental study design with a questionnaire before, immediately after, 1 and 3 months after the intervention. Semi-structured interviews conducted 1 year after the intervention explored participants' opinions and experiences with the intervention and strategies	

(continued)

(continued)

	How to improve program
	• Give outline ahead of time related to topic and expectations of what will happen during workshop • Make it part of something that is already happening (e.g. quarterly CME meetings); give incentives/encourage providers to RSVP to ensure participation • Location/Time: offer workshop on a weekday evening rather than Saturday morning; larger practices throughout town; include in TCHP Grand Rounds (part of CME program) • Make it innovative: new formats, real patients, real scenarios • Present this program to ancillary clinic staff
Results: Of 329 physicians invited, only 13 (3.9%) participated. Participants' mean knowledge score increased from 59.2% to 80% (p < 0.001) but was lower at 3 months (63.3, p < 0.005). Reported awareness of health literacy issues increased from 23.1 to 92.3% (p < 0.001) and remained high at 3 months. *Using simple language, limiting amount of information* and *checking for understanding* were strategies reportedly still used at 3 months. Information presented was new for participants and increased their awareness of communication problems. Health literacy strategies were reportedly simple to use **Conclusions:** Our program increased participants' awareness of health literacy issues and self-reported use of health literacy strategies for communication up to 3 months after the intervention. Future research areas should include replication with a larger sample size, objective measurement of strategies utilized by providers, and measuring patients' opinions about these strategies	**Opinions on content** • Information presented was "eye-opener" • Communication is more than translation or speaking same language • Literacy/health literacy problem is more prevalent than what was thought • Overall, health literacy strategies were well received because they were simple things that could be done in the office • One participant felt strategies were 'basic things' that participant reportedly was already doing, but that would be easy to implement if not using them already **Strategies participants reported using in their practice** • Teach back: simple and works well, took time to implement at first because of the need to remember, but then easy to use, helped to identify words that patients had difficulty understanding • Avoiding medical jargon: difficult to change medical words into something patients can understand, challenging to find simple words for medical terms • Using pictures or models: easy to explain patients the illness and the treatment plan, models is available from pharmaceutical representatives • Slow down when talking with patients: to help with understanding when giving information • Handouts: often use medical terms, one participant became more selective of what they give out to patients, participant found useful to highlight important information, help patients remember what was said in the visit, sometimes end up in trash 'but at least we've tried'

(continued)

(continued)

Participants were asked to express their opinion about the program:	Participants were asked about the actual health literacy strategies discussed during the workshop and their experience with using these in practice:
Participant:	*Participant:*
… sometimes we're practicing medicine so fast and I mean, I don't know about some of my colleagues, but I find that my office staff and myself, sometimes we're like chasing each other… And sometimes I'll even say, "Oh, did I even answer the patient correctly?" And so, going to something like this… made us stop and re-evaluate what we were doing. And the second thing, it gave us some easy things that we could do in our office. It wasn't like you asked me to go out and buy an MRI machine… It was a simple, "Ask the patient, did they understand?" Have them come back to you and explain what you just told them. Or something as simple as [using] a bunch of models…	*It was probably hard to incorporate it because I would have to remember…so at first, it did take a little longer, but then I think my patients taught me some of the stuff, some of the words, again I think it's the words that the patients confuse or the patients don't understand. You know, what words were good, what words were not so good, and then what words were bad, I mean as far as the patient… And for them to walk away and say, "Now, what did I have?"*
Participant:	*Participant:*
I think everything was fine. It was just that I thought maybe there will be some specific guidelines which I didn't' get, you know. They were just average rules and regulations of how to deal with patients and how to get the proper history and communicate with the family and all that, but nothing specific. These are basic things that we already do	*Well, I remember some of the things that ya'll talked about I was already doing. One is to provide handouts in a semi readable format… We do sometimes find them in the trash, but at least we've tried. Sometimes I slow down a little more as far as how quickly I talk*
	Participant:
	We made the language as simple and as everyday as possible, and we do that. We already [did] that. In fact, I never use complicated terms even with the educated patients…

Text Box 2: Texas Childrens' Health Plan Implementation Project: "Can We Do It?"

Connelly, RA, Tran, XG, Xu, L, Giardino, AP, Turner, TL (2014). Increased Use of Health Literacy Strategies for Communication by Physicians. *Health Behavior & Policy Review.* 2014;1(6):460–471

Abstract	Health Literacy Communication Strategies Training Session Content

Objective: About 8 out of 10 parents lack proficient health literacy skills, thereby putting their children at risk for health risks. Physicians do not often use communication strategies that bridge this health literacy gap. This paper describes the effects of a health literacy curriculum on community physicians' knowledge and self-reported use of health literacy communication strategies in pediatric outpatient settings **Methods:** We developed a 3-h active-learning Continuing Medical Education (CME) program using evidence-based teaching strategies for practice change, principles of adult learning theory, and Kolb's model of experiential learning. A 16-item questionnaire assessed health literacy knowledge and self-reported use of six communication strategies at four points in time: immediately before and after, 1 and 3 months following the CME program **Results:** Of physicians completing pre- and post-intervention questionnaires, the average change in use of communication techniques from baseline was 22.6% (11.54–36.89%). A sub-analysis of 28 individuals completing all four study questionnaires revealed most (58–100%) used communication techniques "most of the time" or "always" at 3 months post-intervention. 'Limit Information and Repeat' was the strategy with significantly higher reported use 1 and 3 months after CME. Health literacy knowledge did not change significantly over time **Conclusion:** Our brief, skills-based CME program using evidence-based educational principles and health literacy communication strategies increased community physicians' self-reported use of at least three health literacy communication skills	1. **Introduction and Background (30 min)**
	   a. Parental stories of what it is like to have low health literacy and its impact on their child's health outcomes (video and paper cases), followed by participant reflection
	   b. Didactic
	      i. Definition of health literacy
	      ii. Extent of the problem
	      iii. You can't tell by looking
	      iv. Consequences of low health literacy on health outcomes
	      v. The effects of low health literacy on patient-doctor communication
	   c. Experiential exercise demonstrating what it is like having low health literacy
	2. **Communication gaps and patient safety (35 min)**
	   a. Reflection using a parental video narrative and a paper clinical case
	   b. Didactic
	      i. Health literacy and its impact on medication error and adherence
	      ii. Health literacy and adverse drug events
	      iii. Numeracy—a hidden problem
	      iv. Techniques to minimize medication error and enhance adherence
	         1. Brown bag review
	         2. Minimize complexity
	         3. Provide standardized instruments and dosage tools
	         4. Consider common pitfalls with over-the-counter medications and counsel accordingly
	   c. Small group discussion and large group report out on the question: "How do you enhance patient adherence and improve medication safety in your own practice?"
	3. **Break and allow for questions (10 min)**

(continued)

(continued)

4. Strategies for Communication (25 min)
a.   Reflection using parental video narrative and large group discussion
b.   Didactic session on health literacy communication strategies found to be effective
   i.   Avoid medical jargon
   ii. Check for understanding (Teach Back/Show Me Techniques)
   iii. Encourage parents to ask questions
   iv. Limit the amount of information
   v.   Use pictures or models
   vi. Use patient education handouts effectively
5. Practice with peer-feedback using common pediatric clinical scenarios through role-play (60 min)
a.   Scenario 1 (strategies 1, 2, 3, and 4 above): streptococcal throat infection and management
b.   Scenario 2 (strategies 1, 2, 3, and 4 above): asthma exacerbation in a child with mild persistent asthma with acute bacterial pneumonia
c.   Scenario 3 (all 6 strategies): discussion of the need for a voiding cystourethrogram
6. Action Plan and Questions (10 minutes)
a.   List 3 things you learned during the workshop
b.   With regard to communication with patients, what will you do differently as a result of your participation in this workshop?
c.   In the next month, list ONE strategy you will use to better communicate with your patients.
d.   In the next 3 months, what will you do to improve communication with your patients?

Figure 3
Of the Physicians Who Answered all Surveys, the Percentage Who Self-reported Using Technique Most or All of the Time at Baseline, 1 and 3 months (N = 28 physicians)

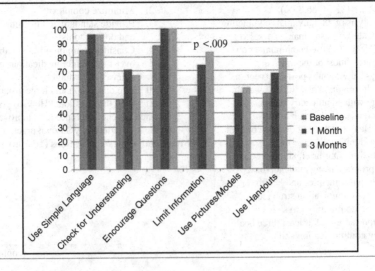

However, the lack of overall progress in increasing health care providers' adoption of these vital behaviors confirms that just putting evidence out there and just "telling" health care providers to do better is not sufficient to change behavior. Instead, education (i.e., telling) of providers needs to be coupled with experiential learning and this harkens back although in a different context to Schwartz and Axelrad's summary described above where education alone is necessary but not sufficient in changing health literacy and instead both educational and behavioral used together were found to be the most effective [8].

One other aspect of the influence model that deserves attention is related to the concept of positive deviance, essentially learning from the individuals and organizations that are demonstrating the desired changed behaviors. Morrison et al. completed a systematic review in which one of the research questions assessed interventions aimed at parents likely to have low health literacy and emergency department use [11]. The interventions and the learnings are summarized below in Table 7.3.

Yin's Educationally Sensitive Patient Outcome (ESPOs) [13]: A Conceptual Model for a Health Literacy

Pediatricians and other health care providers need to have the opportunity to practice communication techniques and receive feedback on their skills from actual and even standardized patients. Training should begin early in medical school and progress through residency and fellowship, as learners provide a large amount of care within the health care system. Additionally, the Accreditation Council of Continuing Medical Education (ACCME) has proposed a menu of criteria for continuing medical education (CME) providers to meet in order to receive 'accreditation with commendation' of which includes patient/public engagement with CME planning and developing communication skills [14]. The ACCME has recognized that it is not enough to include the standard but they have also included that one must have an objective way to measure and provide feedback to the learners on their skills.

Maintenance of Certification, although controversial, also provides a natural platform to implement health literacy strategies and measure system performance and patient outcomes. The American Board of Pediatrics has a performance improvement module focused on health literacy (see Table 7.2, Chap. 6). In 2015, The American Academy of Pediatrics has begun to conduct CME activities which include quality improvement in pediatric practice into their live offerings, of which one program at the annual meeting was centered on enhancing health literacy skills [14, 15]. These innovative programs are designed to help physicians keep abreast of advances in their fields, develop better practice systems, and demonstrate a commitment to lifelong learning while at the same time improve patient outcomes. Asch et al. have provided initial evidence that the quality of medical education influences patient outcomes [16].

Yin et al. have proposed a framework to study this relationship through the use of 'Educationally Sensitive Patient Outcomes' or ESPOs [13]. They state "Providers can be trained to adopt a 'universal precautions approach' to addressing patient health literacy, through the acquisition of specific skills (e.g. teach-back, 'chunk and check' the information, use of plain language written materials) and by learning

Table 7.3 LL interventions to change ED use in populations likely to have LHL

Study	Year	Study design	Control group	Population	Type of intervention	Intervention	Measure of ED use	ED use outcome	Study quality
General health interventions									
Herman [12]	2009	NRCT	Pre- vs postintervention	Primarily low income, minority population; ED nonurgent (triage levels 4–5) patients	Health aid book	"What To Do When Your Child Gets Sick" (3rd–5th grade reading level) and instruction on use of the book	Parent report	30% reduction in number of participants using ED in last 6 months ($P < .0001$)	Good
Herman	2010	NRCT	Pre- vs postintervention	Head Start population, majority Medicaid or uninsured	Health aid book	"What To Do When Your Child Gets Sick" (3rd–5th grade reading level) and instruction on use of the book	Parent report	58% reduction in ED visits per year per child ($P < .001$)	Good
Rector	1999	RCT	No education	Urban Medicaid beneficiaries; ED visit in previous 6 months	Health aid book	Mailed "First Look" (4th grade reading level) to participants	Medicaid records	No difference in ED visits for children whose parent received the intervention	Good
Yoffe	2011	NRCT	Pre- vs postintervention and comparable clinic site	Primarily low income patients	Health aid book	Education booklet, "The pediatric after-hours non-life-and-death almost-an-emergency booklet," addressing most common pediatric ailments with (6th grade reading level) given in primary care clinic	Medical record review	Clinic patients where the booklet were distributed used the ED less ($P < .001$) compared to control clinic patients	Fair

Asthma interventions

Bryant-Stephens	2009	RCT	Randomized crossover design with immediate and delayed intervention	Primarily minority and low income families; child with asthma and controller medication	Home visits with LL course, environmental intervention	Lay health educator home visits using "You Can Control Asthma" curriculum (5th grade reading level) and environmental intervention to avoid triggers	Hospital database	30% reduction in mean ED visits per year per participant ED visits ($P < .001$)	Good
Butz	2006	RCT	Standard asthma education	Primarily minority, low income, and Medicaid patients; child with persistent asthma	Home visits with LL course	Asthma nurse specialist home visits for a 6-months asthma education intervention based on Wee Wheezers and A+ Asthma club programs (3rd–5th grade reading level)	Parent report	18% reduction in ED use ($P < .05$) for 1 or more visits. No difference in mean number of visits.	Good

Morrison, A.K., Myrvik, M.P., Brousseau, D.C., Hofmann, R.G., Stanley, R.M. (2013). The Relationship Between Parent Health Literacy and Pediatric Emergency Department Utilization: A Systematic Review. Academic Pediatrics, 13(5), pp 426–427 [11]

how to take action to improve the 'health literacy environment'." See Fig. 7.1 for a visually representation of this conceptual model. These ESPOs provide a platform for medical education outcomes research and can provide meaningful guidance for health policy.

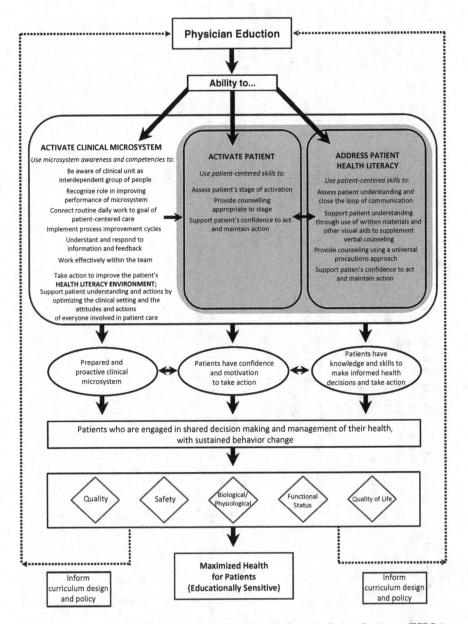

Fig. 7.1 Conceptual model of a health literacy Educationally Sensitive Patient Outcomes (ESPOs). Yin HS, Jay M, Maness L, Zabar S, Kalet A. Health literacy: an educationally sensitive patient outcome. Journal of General Internal Medicine. 2015 Sep 1;30(9):1363–8 (used with permission) [13]

Healthcare cannot really advance without providers letting their patients help themselves and be a *full* partner in making the decisions that affect them. Emma Hill, the editor of Lancet has said: *"Every patient is an expert in their own chosen field, namely themselves and their own life."* Patient-centered care is the bedrock of high quality healthcare delivery. The Institute of Medicine defines patient-centered care as "respecting and responding to patients' wants needs and preferences so that patients can make choices in their care that best fit their individual circumstances" [7]. Patients and families should be empowered to express their healthcare expectations, and health information must be shared in a manner that facilitates understanding. The construct of health literacy is intimately intertwined with patient activation and engagement (Yin). To provide the highest quality care with the best patient outcomes, we must move towards viewing the patient as an individual active participant in his or her care (Fig. 7.1).

The Model for Improvement

"Most people at one time or another have thought about trying to do something better. It might be at home or at work, in recreation or business, for friends or customers. Thinking about doing something better is often easy; actually making a change usually is not." (p.15)

—Langely et al.'s (1996; 2009) Model for Improvement [15, 17]

The Model for Improvement consists of three focusing questions followed by a trial and learning methodology often called the Plan-Do-Study-Act (PDSA) cycle [16]. The Model for Improvement is essentially universally accepted in health care as a valuable tool to promote quality improvement and change efforts. According to its authors, it is easily understood, it can be widely applied to a broad range of situations and circumstances and its application is typically straightforward after minimal orientation and training [17].

The first question relates to the aim of what we are trying to improve and is "what are we trying to accomplish." The second question describes the measurement that we will use to gain feedback on how the change is going and is "how will we know that a change is an improvement?" And, the third question relates to the process or behavior that we will actually change to improve something and the PDSA cycle then trials the change prior to implementation and is "what change can we make that will result in improvement?" The three questions form the element of the model that homes in on the *why* of the change or quality improvement effort, whereas the PDSA cycle zeroes in on the *what* and the *how* of the trial and learning element of the model.

How formal to design a quality improvement effort and with what precision should the measurements be to gauge success or failure of a change to cause improvement is described as a continuum that can be seen as moving from the relatively trivial to the very important. The level of formality and precision progressively increases along this continuum from less formal/precise for the minor issues to more formal/precise for the major or changes [10]. While the processes underpinning the change effort can slide to and fro in terms of formality and precision, the measurements must always be accurate and the commitment to achieving improved quality should be consistent.

Langley et al. are quick to point out that the PDSA cycle is often misused as an implementation of a solution already decided upon and instead, they challenge innovators to use the PDSA to trail targeted and change to learn about this change's impact on the system prior to moving towards implementation in a local context [17]. Central to the functioning of the PDSA cycle is the focus on measurement and action. The actions are based on the review of the measurements in the study phase. Once the measurements determine that the changes are having the desired improvement effect then the implementation process can be undertaken to anchor the new processes or behaviors into routine practice.

The Model for Improvement can be readily applied to health literacy promotion efforts in many contexts. In the health care setting the best practices that are promoted within the use of the universal precautions approach to health literacy are ideal techniques and process changes that can be trialed using the PDSA cycle and once piloted and appropriately modified then can be moved to implementation in the clinical setting (Fig. 7.2).

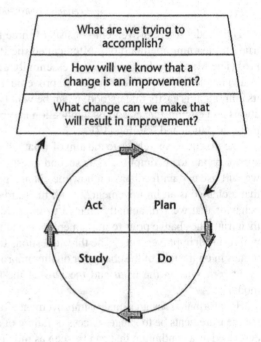

Fig. 7.2 The model for improvement. *Langley, G. J., Moen, R. D., Nolan, K. M., Nolan, T. W., Norman, C. L., & Provost, L. P. (2009). The improvement guide: A practical approach to enhancing organizational performance. 2nd edition. San Francisco, CA: Jossey-Bass. Page 24 (Used with permission)* [17]

What are we trying to accomplish?

How will we know that a change is an improvement?

What change can we make that will result in improvement?

Act   Plan

Study   Do

Sustainability and Spread

The Institute for Healthcare Improvement (IHI) uses straightforward language to define sustainability as locking in the progress made and continually building upon that progress and in a similar manner defines spread as actively disseminating best practice and knowledge about every intervention, and implementing each intervention in every available care setting (5 Million Lives Campaign, 2008). Spread within an organization involves communication and learning for the exchange of knowledge and experience on targeted work practices, expected results, improvement processes, and development of the intervention. The related term, dissemination, is the spread of innovation that is planned, formal and centralized that occurs through vertical hierarchies.

As depicted in Fig. 7.3, Fleiszer and colleagues frame sustainability as multi-dimensional and multi-factorial concept that is ideally viewed as having three characteristics and a set of four preconditions all drawn from their comprehensive concept analysis [2]. The characteristics are (1) benefits, (2) routinization/institutionalization and (3) development. Briefly, the benefits characteristic to sustainability relates to the idea that only effective and valuable innovations should be sustained.

There are two perspectives when considering the benefit characteristic, namely (1) objective, quantifiable results that formally confirm the achievement of an outcome; and (2) subjective, perceived value that is more informal in nature that confirm the positive results to involved stakeholders.

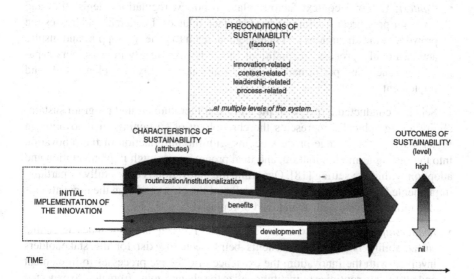

Fig. 7.3 Graphical representation of concept analysis for the sustainability of healthcare innovations. From Fleiszer, A.R. Semenic, S.E., Ritchie, J.A., Richer, M., & Denis, J-L. (2015). The sustainability of healthcare innovations: A concept analysis. Journal of Advanced Nursing, 71(7), 1484–1498 [2] (Used with permission)

The routinization/institutionalization characteristic refers to the adoption of practices that indicate that the innovation has moved from "new" to "accepted" and its structures and processes are now woven in to the fabric of a given setting. In the clinical setting this embedding process would be referred to as being accepted as a standard of care or as a best practice.

Development as a characteristic of sustainability describes the sense of ownership of the innovation by the stakeholders who invest in the ongoing study and enhancement of the initial innovation and addresses the need to apply the innovation in continually evolving environments that require renewal, reinvention and resilience. The ability to adjust and refine an innovation allows the stakeholders to recognize that the ideas and improvements are ultimately their own. The recognition that development can occur only furthers enhances the notion of ownership and the desire to invest and reinvest in maintaining or sustaining the change process.

In addition to characteristics that are essential to an innovation being sustained, Fleiszer and colleagues articulate four preconditions that influence the sustainability as *innovation, context, leadership*, and *processes* [2].

- *Innovation*: Briefly, the innovation precondition relates to aspects of the innovation itself and can best be summarized as the fit with the mission and it's being relevant towards addressing the need or solving the problem. The precondition related to context speaks to both internal and external aspects of a given setting. Internal context factors deal with organizational culture and project management capacity to keep an innovation on track [2].
- *Context*: External context factors relate to policy, regulations, legislation and financial pressures (funding or market place related). Leadership addresses the prowess of the champions and management team to generate support and inspire action. Finally, process preconditions look a lot like quality improvement capabilities such as performance monitoring and ability to plan, trial and implement.

Scheirer conducted a review of the empirical literature around program sustainability and graphically represents the chronology of sustaining an innovation in Fig. 7.4 where the change process begins with the introduction of the innovation into the setting termed, initiation, and then progresses through implementation and adoption within the setting [18]. Over time the innovation is either fully or partially implemented as determined by an evaluation of the effort and then the innovation is seen to either be sustained, abandoned or replaced.

- *Leadership and Processes*: Both Scheirer and Fleiszer and colleagues agree that sustainability is hinged on benefits being seen to exist for the stakeholders involved with the innovation, the existence of effective processes to implement and ultimately routinize or institutionalize the change going from new to expected practice, and the existence of some level of flexibility such that unique contextual aspects can be recognized and accommodated [2, 18]. In addition, both authors recognize the need for leadership in the form of a champion for a given innovation as well as the need for the innovation to fit within the mission of the stakeholders as well.

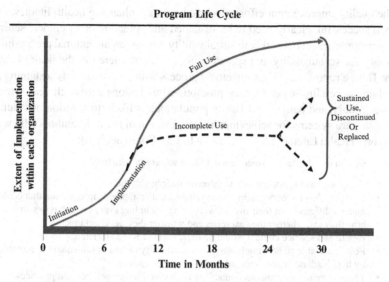

Fig. 7.4 Implementation of an innovation and possibility of sustained use *(Used with permission from Scheirer, 2005)* [18]

Scheirer and colleagues specifically draws attention to the observation that innovations may be either fully or partially implemented over time. A number of factors affect the extent to which an innovation is fully implemented and she specifically calls for the use specific evaluation methods and tools such as a logic model to assist in defining the components of the innovation that are essential towards achieving the desired outcome.

Linking her work on sustainability to the field of implementation science, Scheirer addresses the notion of spread or dissemination as an important dimension after an innovation is sustained in its original setting. Spread, essentially the adoption of the innovation beyond its original implementation site can occur in a variety of ways. Buchanan and colleagues offer the idea of spread occurring across a continuum moving from copying the innovation exactly as it was previously implemented to the other extreme where the original innovation serves only as a guiding framework for action in the new setting [2].

These distinctions become important to the improvement leader since understanding the nuances of the innovation that is to be sustained or "hardwired" and then spreading that to other colleagues or units throughout the setting is ideally done from a position of knowledge and understanding. Having one's conceptual frameworks clearly in mind and recognizing the multiple factors at play in a complex environment can help facilitate change and confront barriers or resistance. Finally, Buchanan, Fitzgerald, and Ketley from the UK add to this discussion taking on a more ecological or systems based approach looking and describe at the levels that change occurs which can be simplified in healthcare for this discussion as, change and adoption of innovation occurring at the (1) individual, (2) unit and (3) across organization levels [3].

The quality improvement efforts designed around enhancing health literacy, once deemed successful, clearly need to be sustained and spread to other clinical settings. The characteristics associated with sustainability and the organizational preconditions necessary for sustainability and spread ought to be considered in the health literacy arena. Thus, a robust quality improvement process with an eye towards sustaining and spreading successful health literacy promoting innovations across clinical settings, provider groups and patient and family populations is likely to position our patients and health care systems for achieving the stated vision of the IOM authors who wrote the report "Health Literacy: A Prescription to End Confusion" [6]:

"We believe a health-literate America would be a society in which:

- Everyone has the opportunity to improve their health literacy.
- Everyone has the opportunity to use reliable, understandable information that could make a difference in their overall well-being, including everyday behaviors such as how they eat, whether they exercise, and whether they get checkups.
- Health and science content would be basic parts of K-12 curricula.
- People are able to accurately assess the credibility of health information presented by health advocate, commercial, and new media sources.
- There is monitoring and accountability for health literacy policies and practices.
- Public health alerts, vital to the health of the nation, are presented in everyday terms so that people can take needed action.
- The cultural contexts of diverse peoples, including those from various cultural groups and non-English-speaking peoples, are integrated in to all health information.
- Health practitioners communicate clearly during all interactions with their patients, using everyday vocabulary.
- There is ample time for discussions between patients and healthcare providers.
- Patients feel free and comfortable to ask questions as part of the healing relationship.
- Rights and responsibilities in relation to health and health care are presented or written in clear, everyday terms so that people can take needed action.
- Informed consent documents used in health care are developed so that all people can give or withhold consent based on information they need and understand."

Institute of Medicine (U.S.). Committee on Health Literacy. & Nielsen-Bohlman, L. (2004). *Health literacy: A prescription to end confusion*. Washington, D.C.: National Academies Press. Page 13 (used with permission) [6]

References

1. Wiltsey-Stirman S, Kimberly J, Cook N, Calloway A, Castro F, Charns M. The sustainability of new programs and innovations: a review of the empirical literature and recommendations for future research. Implement Sci. 2012;7:17–35.
2. Fleiszer AR, Semenic SE, Ritchie JA, Richer M, Denis J-L. The sustainability of healthcare innovations: a concept analysis. J Adv Nurs. 2015;71(7):1484–98.
3. Buchanan D, Fitzgerald L, Ketley D. The sustainability and spread of organizational change: modernizing healthcare. London: Routledge; 2007.
4. Parker RM, Ratzan SC, Lurie N. Health literacy: a policy challenge for advancing high-quality health care. Health Aff. 2003;22(4):147–53.

5. Koh HK, Berwick DM, Clancy CM, Baur C, Brach C, Harris LM, Zerhusen EG. New federal policy initiatives to boost health literacy can help the nation move beyond the cycle of costly 'crisis care'. Health Aff. 2012 Jan;18:10–377.

6. IOM. Health literacy: a prescription to end confusion. Washington: The National Academies Press; 2004.

7. Chao S, Anderson K, Hernandez L, editors. Toward health equity and patient-centeredness: integrating health literacy, disparities reduction, and quality improvement: workshop summary. Washington: National Academies Press; 2009.

8. Schwartz DD, Axelrad MA. Healthcare partnerships for pediatric adherence: promoting collaborative management for pediatric chronic illness care. Switzerland: Springer; 2015.

9. Patterson K, Grrnny J, Maxfield D, McMillan R, Switzler A. Influencer: the power to change anything. New York: McGraw Hill; 2008.

10. Bandura A. Personal interview with authors Patterson K, Grrnny J, Maxfield D, McMillan R, Switzler A (2008). Influencer: the power to change anything. New York: McGraw Hill; 2006.

11. Morrison AK, Myrvik MP, Brousseau DC, Hofmann RG, Stanley RM. The relationship between parent health literacy and pediatric emergency department utilization: a systematic review. Acad Pediatr. 2013;13(5):426–7.

12. Personal correspondence June 9, 2016, American Academy of Pediatrics Committee on Continuing Medical Education.

13. Yin HS, Jay M, Maness L, Zabar S, Kalet A. Health literacy: an educationally sensitive patient outcome. J Gen Intern Med. 2015;30(9):1363–8.

14. Accreditation Council of Continuing Medical Education. Proposal for a menu of new criteria for accreditation with commendation. 2016. http://www.accme.org/sites/default/files/718_20160112_Proposal_for_a_Menu_of_New_Criteria_for_Accreditation_with_Commendation.pdf. Accessed 28 June 2016.

15. Langley GJ, Nolan KM, Nolan TW, Norman CL, Provost LP. The improvement guide: a practical approach to enhancing organizational performance. San Francisco: Jossey-Bass; 1996.

16. Asch DA, Nicholson S, Srinivas SK, Herrin J, Epstein AJ. How do you deliver a good obstetrician? Outcome-based evaluation of medical education. Acad Med. 2014;89(1):24–6.

17. Langley GJ, Moen RD, Nolan KM, Nolan TW, Norman CL, Provost LP. The improvement guide: a practical approach to enhancing organizational performance. 2nd ed. San Francisco: Jossey-Bass; 2009.

18. Scheirer MA. Is sustainability possible? A review and commentary on empirical studies of program sustainability. Am J Eval. 2005;26:320–47.

Index

Printed in the United States
By Bookmasters